# The Heart Treasure
## of *Taijiquan*

太極拳行法釋要

# The Heart Treasure
## of *Taijiquan*

太極拳行法釋要

Written and Spoken by Ren Gang
Translated and Edited by Mattias Daly

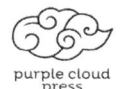

Copyright © 2021 by Mattias Daly
All rights reserved under International and Pan-American Copyright Conventions

ISBN-13: 9798667766766

Library of Congress Control Number
2020924552

Front Cover Image: "Xuanwu, God of the North,"
Attributed to Bai Liangyu (白良玉, fl. ca. 1195-1124 CE),
Washington, DC: Freer Gallery of Art/Arthur M. Sackler Gallery

The image "Shang Dynasty Bronze Vessel" on page 52 is from the collection of the National Palace Museum, Taipei, Taiwan, Republic of China. Other images come from the author's private collection or the public domain.

*Cover design by Anne-Maree Taranto (contact@rhapsodica.com) and Mattias Daly*
*Interior design by Barbara Tada (www.pixelgardendesign.com)*

Published by Purple Cloud Press
purplecouldinstitute.com
purplecloudpress@gmail.com

The author and the publisher of this book are not responsible for any harm resulting from use of the methods described in this book. We advise readers to seek instruction from a knowledgeable taijiquan teacher in person. We also advise readers to consult with a licensed healthcare professional before embarking upon a new course of physical training.

No part of this book may be reproduced or used in any form or by any means, electronic or mechanical, including photocopying, scanning, recording, or by any information storage and retrieval system, without prior written permission from the publisher. If you come across a bootleg version of this book and benefit from it, please consider buying a real copy. A translation such as this one takes many hundreds of hours of painstaking work to produce, and can only be undertaken after years of practice and thousands of hours of study. Readers' support is deeply appreciated, as well as key to making further translations possible!

"Very well written and well researched, with just the right balance of personal input and academic disinterest. Mattias Daly is a passionate young man searching for answers. Fluent in Mandarin, he spent many years in China studying with masters of internal Chinese martial arts, with all the ups and downs that such a process entails. As a result, this book is both straightforward and insightful, both logical and full of hope, a refreshingly commonsense approach to both the secrets and practical realities of the Chinese martial traditions.

A must-read for practitioners of Yang-style tai chi chuan and all those interested in the philosophy of Chinese martial arts in general."

— Kostas Dervenis,
Headmaster of the Pammachon Cultural Foundation,
author of *The Martial Arts of Ancient Greece* and *The Magus of Java*

"Perhaps the best book translated into English on the real practice of Taijiquan and what it takes to learn it. Within its pages is also the best elucidation of the Taiji Classic, returning the words to their rightful place as a practical guide to developing skill and not the esoteric text so many make it out to be."

— Andrew Nugent-Head,
Founder of the Association for Traditional Studies,
Chinese medicine physician and educator,
and practitioner of Yin style *baguazhang*

# Purple Cloud's Vision

Purple Cloud Press was founded upon the premise that theoretical knowledge and practical experience must be accrued in tandem in order for people to gain profound insights into the nuances of classical writings. All Purple Cloud Press publications are written and translated by scholar-physicians and scholar-practitioners in pursuit of the following threefold mission:

- To publish the works of the founders of the Purple Cloud Institute as well as other authors' writings in the fields of Eastern medicine, Asian spiritual traditions, and martial arts;
- To translate ancient foundational texts from Asian languages into English;
- To commission original writings on masters' and teachers' lineage-based traditions.

Purple Cloud Press incentivizes authors and translators by guaranteeing them a large percentage of royalties in order to encourage continued translation projects, as well as by providing a platform to reach the broadest possible readership. Purple Cloud Press strongly believes that our efforts will greatly increase the English-speaking world's access to the profundity of formerly unavailable treasures.

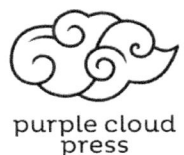

太極是讓人們通向身心健康的一條光明大道。
願大家和我一起領略一路上的美景！

任剛

    *Taiji is a bright path that leads those who walk it towards health in body and mind.*
*May we enjoy the beautiful views along this road together!*

*R.G.*

# Contents

Martial Prowess and Magnanimity
    Foreword by Cai Songfang . . . . . . . . . . . . . . . . . . . . . . . . . . . . . xi
*Taijiquan's* Thoroughly Modern Inheritor
    Foreword by He Jihong . . . . . . . . . . . . . . . . . . . . . . . . . . . . . . . xv
When Martial Arts Merge with the Dao
    Foreword by Huo Zhenhuan . . . . . . . . . . . . . . . . . . . . . . . . . . xxi
Ultimate Truths Are Inexpressible; Sages' Minds Are Limitless . . . xxv
Destined for *Taijiquan* – Author's Preface . . . . . . . . . . . . . . . . . . xxix
Notes on the English Edition – Translator's Introduction. . . . . . . . . 1
Chapter 1: On Culture. . . . . . . . . . . . . . . . . . . . . . . . . . . . . . . . . . . .11
    Putting Chinese culture into practice via *taijiquan* . . . . . . . . . . . .11
    Do you treat your culture like a son, or like a pig? . . . . . . . . . . . 15
Chapter 2: On Training . . . . . . . . . . . . . . . . . . . . . . . . . . . . . . . . . 19
    Prerequisite knowledge for successful *taijiquan* practice:
        On "qi" and "Qi" . . . . . . . . . . . . . . . . . . . . . . . . . . . . . . . . . . 19
    The three indispensable factors in *taijiquan* practice:
        A destination, a vessel, and a way to power your vessel. . . . . . . 23
Chapter 3: Martial Theory. . . . . . . . . . . . . . . . . . . . . . . . . . . . . . . 27
    Explaining the key points in Wang Zongyue's
        *Treatise on Taijiquan* . . . . . . . . . . . . . . . . . . . . . . . . . . . . . . 27
    Wang Zongyue's original text. . . . . . . . . . . . . . . . . . . . . . . . . . . 27
    An explanation of the *Treatise on Taijiquan*. . . . . . . . . . . . . . . . . 29
Chapter 4: Dispelling Doubts . . . . . . . . . . . . . . . . . . . . . . . . . . . . 67
Chapter 5: Resolving Confusion . . . . . . . . . . . . . . . . . . . . . . . . . .111
Chapter 6: Elucidations . . . . . . . . . . . . . . . . . . . . . . . . . . . . . . . . 153
    Some thoughts on traditional Chinese martial arts. . . . . . . . . . . 153
    On "force" . . . . . . . . . . . . . . . . . . . . . . . . . . . . . . . . . . . . . . . . . 156
    The *guqin*, the game of go, calligraphy, and painting. . . . . . . . . . 157
    *Taijiquan's* deepest teaching: Making use of emptiness. . . . . . . . 159
Chapter 7: The Cat's Marvelous Methods
    Original text and commentary . . . . . . . . . . . . . . . . . . . . . . . . . 165

Part 1 ............................................................ 167
Part 2 ............................................................ 168
Part 3 ............................................................ 177
Part 4 ............................................................ 185
Part 5 ............................................................ 196
Real *Taijiquan* – Afterword by Wang Xiaopeng ................. 201
The Shining Path – Afterword by Zhong Yingyang.............. 207
Appendix – Guide to Chinese names mentioned in the text....... 213
Other Publications by Purple Cloud Press ..................... 216

# Martial Prowess and Magnanimity

## *Foreword by Cai Songfang*

I FIRST MET Ren Gang in 1987. Years fly by, and in the blink of an eye we've known each other for more than three decades. When we first met he was still a young lad who'd just started to learn martial arts, practicing *taijiquan* and push hands with a class full of youthful enthusiasts led by his neighbor, Guo Dadong, in Xiangyang Park. It was always apparent that Ren Gang pursued his martial arts studies with real sincerity. Whether he was practicing forms or push hands, he would always train with remarkable zeal. As a result, not only did he always quickly grasp ahold of what his teachers were trying to convey, he also thought up creative ways to distill the underlying principles. It is hard to say whether he was the smartest among that early group of students, but back then he was definitely the most tenacious, and certainly the most enamored with *taijiquan*.

Fortune was on Ren Gang's side, and it put him into contact with his gracious teacher, the famous *taiji* master Dong Bin. Master Dong held back no secrets, passing the entirety of his lifetime of training experience and realizations to his young pupil. As for Ren, he immersed himself in the search for *taijiquan*'s profound truths. Adept at unraveling conundrums in his mind and dedicated to research, he frequently sought out his teacher to discuss important points from the classic treatises on martial arts, and he also experimented with these points in actual practice. Without a doubt, in those early years Ren Gang found his way into the gate of mystery that lies hidden in the classical writings on martial arts. His *taiji* skills, naturally enough, took a quantum leap.

Perhaps, as the Chinese have long said, the heavens really do look out for those who put their hearts into things. With Dong Bin's detailed instruction and his own tireless efforts over more than a dozen hot summers and cold winters, by 2005 Ren Gang's skills began to match my own. In more recent years, possibly aided by his Buddhist practice, Ren has seen even further into *taijiquan*'s most subtle and recondite principles. His abilities in terms of push hands and actual fighting, having reached somewhere close to the pinnacle, eclipsed mine long ago. Naturally, in today's martial arts world, people who truly comprehend the profundity of *taijiquan* are as rare as phoenix feathers, but Ren Gang is truly a *taiji* dragon!

Along with being skilled with his fists, Ren also has a kind heart. Intimately aware of the intrinsic difficulties of martial arts study, some time ago he made a vow to unreservedly pass on the theories of *taijiquan*, as well as all of his own insights, to all pure-hearted seekers.

Additionally, I have never known Ren Gang to be unduly concerned with questions of lineages and schools. Regardless of whether people practice internal or external martial arts, or Chinese *gongfu* or foreign fighting techniques, so long as their goal is to exchange combat arts and discuss the martial way, then they are welcome to try their hand with him. The majority of those who have come to test their skills against Ren Gang have arrived with hearts full of expectations, and then left fully convinced, with smiles on their faces to boot. With regards to imparting his *taijiquan* inheritance, for years Ren has poured his energy and enthusiasm into grooming disciples in the younger generation. Deeply appreciative of the Buddhist maxim, "the Dharma relies upon people to flourish," he set out to foster ten students who will fully inherit the essence of his teachings. This transmission will lay a foundation from which authentic *taijiquan* knowledge and skills can become widely available.

As one of Ren Gang's elders, I've personally witnessed the effort he has applied to carrying *taijiquan* forward by training the next generation of talented students. This is no easy task. It brings me great happiness, on behalf of the worlds of *taijiquan* and Chinese martial arts at large, to know that there is a teacher in the prime of his life who is at once versed in the classical writings, a capable educator, and qualified to preserve and promote our traditional culture. It is my wish that Ren Gang will obtain ever more profound insights during his quest to plumb *taijiquan*'s mysteries, and that his vows to disseminate *taijiquan* teachings will come to swift fruition!

*Shanghai, 2013*


Cai Songfang is a renowned *taijiquan* and internal martial arts practitioner. He carries the lineage of the great internal martial arts master Ye Dami, from whom he received thorough instruction in four of *taijiquan*'s thirteen forces: *peng, lü, ji,* and *an*. Master Cai's deepest training is in the orthodox Wudang *wuji* methods transmitted within *Yang* family *taijiquan*. Although he only obtained transmission in four of the thirteen forces, his skill is nevertheless superb, particularly in terms of push hands. His application of the mysterious "empty force" skill in push hands is admired around the world.

Master Cai has been influential in the Southeast Asian and North American martial arts worlds. During the 1980s and 90s he accepted numerous invitations to visit the United States to teach fighting techniques and exchange knowledge. When several well-known martial artists from San Francisco sought him out to test their skills, he sent them flying as soon as they touched hands, causing enough of a stir to attract the attention of the local media. Later, when a 300-pound *wing chun* master challenged him in from of TV cameras, Master Cai sent the fellow flying so far and so quickly that he seemed to simply disappear from the camera frame!

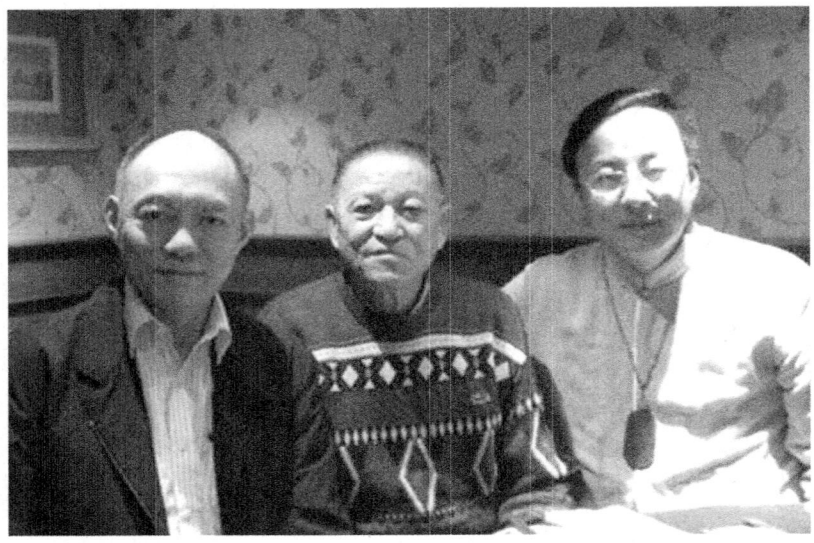

Huo Zhenhuan, Cai Songfang, Ren Gang (left to right)

# Taijiquan's Thoroughly Modern Inheritor

## Foreword by He Jihong

TAIJIQUAN IS AN important part of traditional Chinese culture, and it's also one of the gems of the Chinese martial arts. Its deep philosophical basis, its unexcelled fighting techniques, and its effectiveness in terms of promoting good spirits and good health have earned it well-deserved recognition by Chinese martial arts enthusiasts all around the world.

Although *taijiquan* is ultimately a fighting art, those enthusiasts who are familiar with its underlying philosophy and who've already "entered the door" will no doubt agree that *taijiquan* is not quite the same as other athletic activities. The difference lies not only in the fact that *taijiquan* is something one can study and practice for as long as one lives, but also in the fact that in order to have any hope of success in this art, one needs to cultivate integrity as much as one needs to develop technical skill.

Throughout the course of its long history, numerous renowned *taijiquan* practitioners have written books in which they lay out valuable theories, experiences, and training methods. Consequently, quite a few different lineages have been established, but for various reasons there have long existed degrees of inter-school rivalry and protectionism. As a result, each lineage's theoretical teachings and secret technical instructions have been passed down only through formally inducted disciples, and never through outsiders. Nevertheless, while this custom has led to the development of markedly distinct lineages, they all emphasize the importance of observing and testing the character of their disciples, and they all agree that cultivating integrity comes before martial training. This is because skills will only stand upright where there is a solid foundation of integrity. Additionally, almost without exception, all schools emphasize the value of the master-disciple relationship and chisel martial ethics into their school rules. All of this is done in order to produce lineage holders who possess equal parts virtue and skill.

I became acquainted with Ren Gang in the early 1990s, when Master Cai Songfang brought him to me to practice push hands. This bookish young student of Master Dong Bin was humble, eager to learn, and extremely hardworking. It's well-known that in Shanghai there are two major lineages of Yang family *taijiquan*, one being the Dong line associated with Yue Huanzhi, and the other being the Ye line, represented by Ye Dami. Dong Bin was a highly cultivated *taijiquan* practitioner who inherited teachings directly from Yue Huanzhi and attained the true depths of Yue and Dong Shizuo's transmissions. Yue Huanzhi in particular was the sort of *taijiquan* master who was almost the stuff of legend—his skills far surpassed what's commonly seen in the martial arts world of today.

With the publishing of this book, Ren Gang is fully revealing the secrets of the Dong line of Yang family *taijiquan* to the public. Since not all schools' training methods are the same, I will highlight an indispensable point in Ren's teachings in this introduction: the need to "straighten the waist." Because this way of training is exactly the opposite of the "push out the *mingmen*" instruction common to numerous schools of internal martial arts, many people find it difficult to accept. In the past we all used to push out our *mingmen* regions while training, and believed that if this wasn't done then we were practicing our martial arts incorrectly.[1]

---

[1] The *mingmen*, from "命門," is sometimes translated literally as a the "gate of life." It refers to the region of the body located roughly level with the belly button in the center of the lower back (acupuncture more specifically locates it in the space beneath the second lumbar vertebra), as well as the functions of *qi* that are associated with this location, especially when it is made active through internal martial arts or Daoist cultivation. Because the *mingmen*

I have deep experience with this problem. When I was eighty years old I took Ren's instruction to straighten my waist on board, and after training with this method for ten months I felt like I'd reached a whole new level in my *taiji*. Even Ren Gang was shocked that an old fogey in his eighties could grasp this technique in just ten short months! The fruits of my new way of training were just beginning to bud, but I could already feel that the waist is really and truly the human body's primary seat of control, and that it is from there that the entirety of the body's intent and *qi* are mobilized. This made me think of the some of the things Hao Shaoru[2] described in his book.

Beyond straightening the waist, I learned many other new points of theory and approaches to fighting from Ren Gang's book. That these little-known secrets from Yang style *taijiquan* are now being made public is truly cause for celebration.

Throughout the decades that Ren Gang has devoted to studying martial arts, he has always honored his lineage, looked up to his teachers and elders, treated his peers with kindness, and scrupulously conducted himself in accordance with the code of martial ethics. His comportment is something everybody in this community has noticed. He's not merely possessed of excellent *taijiquan* combat skills. He also has a comprehensive knowledge of *taijiquan* theory, making him the most outstanding up-and-coming master I've met in the last fifty years. He's currently the director of an art gallery devoted to agarwood sculpture and other forms of classical Chinese art, but in spite of his heavy workload he has taken the time to publish this book as a contribution to the Chinese martial arts. As such, as old and grey as I might be, it brings me great pleasure to write this short introduction on his behalf.

*May 31st, 2013*

---

point is located in the center of the lumbar region, it is also often used to refer to the lumbar as a whole, and not simply this particular "acupoint." The *mingmen* will be discussed in detail throughout the book.

[2] Hao Shaoru's book, published in 1963, is called 《武式太極拳》 or *Wu Style Taijiquan*.

Between the years of 1933 and 1960, He Jihong followed Ding Ranqing, a student of Master Ye Dami, in the study of Ye family Yang style *taijiquan*. Subsequently he also trained push hands with the famous Wu style *taijiquan* master, Pei Zuying. In 1966 he was introduced to one of his colleagues' fathers, Master Xu Bingsheng, with whom he studied Tian Zhaolin's large frame Yang style *taijiquan* and push hands. Master Xu was then already nearly eighty years old. In earlier years he had served as Shell Oil's managing director in China, during which time he entreated Master Tian Zhaolin to come to his home for private lessons. Thanks to his excellent progress, Master Tian dubbed him one of his lineage's "five tigers."

Master Xu was also highly skilled in internal *qigong*, which gave him unique insights into the use of intent and *qi* in *taijiquan*. He was even capable of placing his palm atop the head of a stroke victim suffering from hemiplegia and causing the patient's palsied hand to open. Xu never formally accepted any disciples, nor did he teach martial arts in public settings. It was He Jihong's fate to receive more than ten years of selfless instruction from Master Xu—these years were the most important turning point in his lifetime of *taijiquan* study.

Good fortune visited He Jihong again in 1973 when he made acquaintance with another highly accomplished disciple of Master Ye Dami, Jin Renlin. Master Jin was famous for his research into *taijiquan* theory—his contemporaries used to say that he filled his belly not by eating food, but by feasting on classic treatises. He had a comprehensive knowledge of Ye family *taijiquan* which he imparted to Master He, helping He to take another leap forward in his understanding of the principles of this martial art.

Throughout a life dedicated to *taijiquan*, two of the best friends He Jihong has made are Master Wang Zhuanghong and his martial arts brother Xu Yuqi, both of whom he regularly seeks out to practice push hands and exchange fighting techniques. He's friendships with these two modern-day masters have been mutually beneficial. Since the mid-1970s, Master He has been teaching *taijiquan* for free in Xiangyang Park in Shanghai. His friendly and open personality and peaceful way of going about things have allowed him to enjoy a life free of petty conflicts.

In the early 1980s, Master He taught Ye family Yang style *taijiquan* to practitioners in the city of Jiaxing in Zhejiang Province. It remains popular there to this day thanks his student Cai Guangfu, who has carried the tradition forward. Cai Guangfu, who is nationally recognized as a seventh *dan* master, is currently the vice team leader of the Zhejiang Province Martial Arts Experts Group, and chairman of the Jiaxing City Martial Arts Association. He is praised by students and teachers alike for his friendly ways.

Writings on martial techniques by Master He include *Some Modest Opinions Regarding Taijiquan and Taiji Push Hands*, *The Essentials of Taijiquan Push Hands Training*, *Reflections Upon My Experiences with Movement Forms*, *A Discussion on the Rotations and Revolutions in Taijiquan Forms*, *A Treatise on the Source of Life and Mind in the Lumbar Crevice*, and *How to Train in Wudang Ye Family Taijiquan*.

Master He's *taijiquan* forms are characterized by lightness, agility, and tranquility. His external stances are elegant and erect, while his internal *qi* is boundless. When pushing hands he guides his opponent with his spirit and *qi*, and uses his muscles and bones merely as complements. He stresses that teachers should never be afraid to learn from their students, that there is no end point on the road of learning, and that regardless of a person's age or generation, so long as the person has aptitude, then that person is worthy of seeking out for advice.

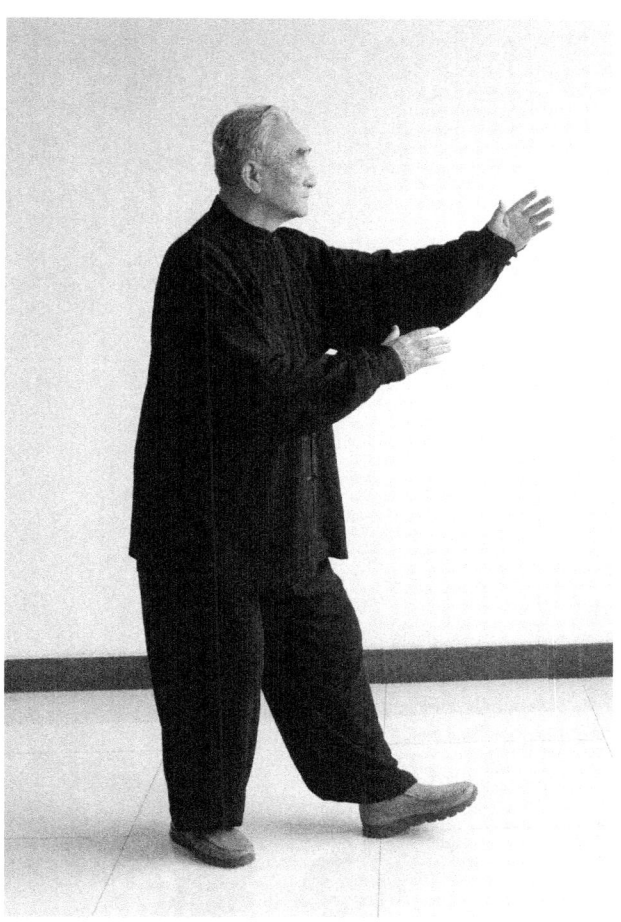

Master He Jihong

# When Martial Arts Merge with the Dao

## Foreword by Huo Zhenhuan

I HAVE LOVED practicing martial arts ever since I was a teenager, but it took me many years before I realized that martial accomplishment is far more than a question of how one moves one's hands and feet or how low or high one's stances are. Rather, a high level martial artist is one who has learned to develop and then *use* his or her latent capabilities, thereby surpassing the commonly-accepted limits of human ability.

For this reason, for the last few years I've been extremely interested in research and dialogue related to martial arts training of a high enough level to transcend the mundane. My interest was initially piqued when I read the term "martial arts lead to the Dao" in one of Master Sun Lutang's[3] books. Later on, I heard about and eventually personally witnessed the use of "empty force," with which one can

---

[3] The phrase in question here reads "拳與道合," which could also be translated as "the studies of martial arts and Dao merge together." This four-character phrase, although widely attributed to Sun Lutang, seems to not come directly from his own writings, and rather from later martial artists' synopses of the great master's written teachings. Thrice in his book *Elucidating the Truths of Martial Arts and Mind* (《拳意述真》 or *Quan Yi Shu Zhen*), Sun uses a phrase written in classical Chinese, "與道合真," to describe the highest pinnacle of martial arts practice. In the rawest possible translation, this Daoist-sounding term reads "with-Dao-merge-real." It refers to a practitioner achieving a state of existence where his or her being has merged with the ultimate nature of reality, or Dao. Some of Sun Lutang's writings have been translated into English and other languages.

repel opponents without even touching them. Having seen empty force firsthand, I was able to lend some credence to legends of people reaching the stage of not needing to see or hear their opponents in order to defend themselves—practitioners who have reached this state are supposedly able to spontaneously strike down attackers who are sneaking up from behind. The development of abilities that are wholly absent in everyday people is a topic I've long sought to understand.

I haven't known Ren Gang for a long time, having sought him out only a few years ago on the strength of Master Cai Songfang's glowing recommendation. Much to my benefit, Master Cai has mentored me since the 1980s. A master of *taijiquan wuji zhanzhuang*, Cai has been able to use mind and *qi* to formlessly repel people for years. Even though he possesses highly refined martial skill, Master Cai remains at heart a humble and tireless student. He described Ren Gang to me as a practitioner who surpasses his teachers, and an accomplished scholar who understands the true principles underlying *taijiquan*.

As a grand-disciple of Grandmaster Yue Huanzhi, Master Ren is a descendant of a renowned lineage and person whose years of intensive study have given him a firm grasp on *taijiquan*'s enigmatic philosophy. The distance between Hong Kong and Shanghai means that we have only met a few short times, but Ren Gang's systematic explanations and demonstrations have allowed me to experience the high-level philosophy of *taijiquan* as a tangible reality. Our meetings have also allowed me to bear witness to the fact that Ren's skill exists at the prior heaven level; that he uses prior heaven *qi* and has transcended training in later heaven *qi*; that he requires his students to reach the stage of unity of the self and all things; and that he teaches martial arts as a straightforward path leading to the Dao. It is a wonderful thing that Master Ren unselfishly offers his priceless insights to the public within these pages. This book will enlighten all those who seek to deepen their knowledge of the martial way, and it will play an important role in raising the stature of the Chinese martial arts in general. I happily recommend this book to all fellow enthusiasts.

*March 13th, 2014*

Master Huo Zhenhuan is a lover of the martial arts who has for years tirelessly taken part in promoting them on the international stage. He is the current director of the Hong Kong Wushu Union, chairman of the Wushu Federation of Asia, and a member of the executive committee of the International Wushu Federation.

Master Huo first encountered the martial arts in his adolescent years. While studying in England he started out training in the Japanese arts of *judo* and *aikido*, and then in university he turned to Yang family *taijiquan* before becoming immersed in *yiquan*[4] and embarking upon decades of exploration of the internal martial arts.

Over the years, Master Huo has received instruction from numerous accomplished masters, including such *taijiquan* teachers as Yang Shouzhong, Cai Songfang, and Feng Zhiqiang. In *yiquan* he has trained with such representatives of the second generation as Han Xinghuan, Yao Zongxun, Han Qiao, Han Sihuang, and Yang Shaogeng. He has also received guidance from many other outstanding members of the martial arts community.

Although Master Huo is generally busy with his work as a public servant, martial arts are fully integrated with his daily life, and he has trained daily for dozens of years.

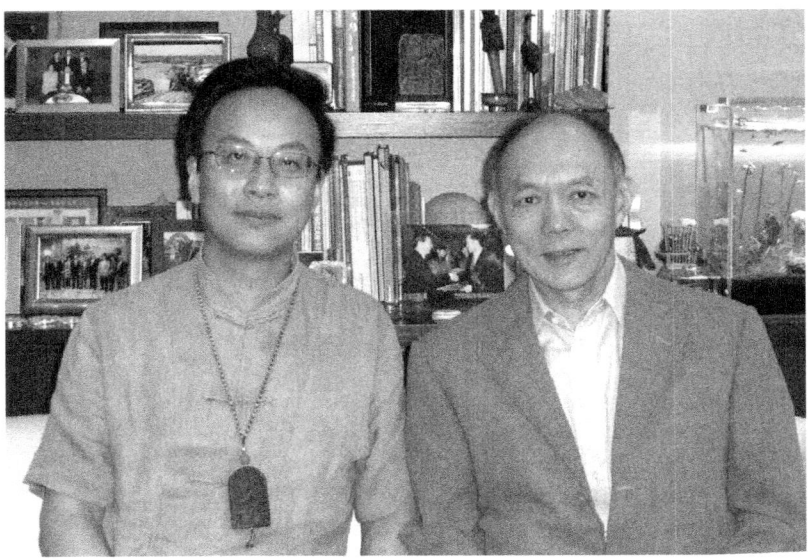

Ren Gang and Huo Zhenhuan

---

[4] Written "意拳," *yiquan* is an internal martial art developed in the twentieth century by Wang Xiangzhai.

# Ultimate Truths Are Inexpressible; Sages' Minds Are Limitless

## *Foreword by Yu Hongkun*

CHAN BUDDHISM RELIES upon direct mind-to-mind transmission; Ren Gang's *taijiquan* is the same. Chan is frequently described as being "a unique teaching beyond the sutras" and "a direct pointing out of the human mind;"[5] similarly, Master Ren's *taijiquan* contains movement that is not apparent, and which is based upon a pure merging of the spirit. In this merging, there exists neither self nor opponent.

When the body moves in non-apparent ways, it is unimpeded and unfettered, and the owner of that body is in no way attached to it. When the spirit is fully merged, it unifies with the opponent's *qi* and then moves it, so there exists neither self nor opponent.

The secret of being so skilled that one has no opponents lies in non-acknowledgement. When there is no acknowledgement of opposition, then there is no resistance, and both individuals engaged in combat simply merge into a single state of *taiji*. The *qi* passing through a fighter's own body unifies with his or her opponent's *qi*, and is thereby both sensed and understood. That's what the *Treatise on Taijiquan* refers to when it states, "Others cannot fathom me—I alone know others. All heroes without match started here."

---

[5] The first phrase is written "經外別傳" and the second as "直指人心." When the depth of their meaning is understood, it is clear that these two pithy sentences at once refer to the essential Chan/Zen teachings, as well as synopsize them.

There are innumerable styles of Chinese martial arts, all of which possess their own wonders. In accordance with the natural diversity of students' innate talents, the arts provide a variety of entry methods for beginners. Some schools start with the physique, some start with strength, some start with *qi*, and some start with intent—there are unique methods designed for training in all of these approaches. However, these ways all fundamentally exist at the level of *doing*, and thus it is easy for students to become lost in the minutiae of their personal training experiences. Methods based upon doing cannot lead people to the highest achievement.

Each and every movement in Master Ren Gang's *taijiquan* is executed while sensing and understanding both his own and others' *shen* and *qi*, such that an opponent has no place to land his or her strength. His execution is a marvelous illustration of the *taijiquan* saying, "A single feather cannot be added, and a gnat finds nowhere to land."

Ren Gang is a modest gentleman, highly cultivated in the timeless manner, and compassionate in his heart. *Taijiquan* is not the only path he walks. It is the collective good fortune of students everywhere that brother Ren Gang is revealing the lost internal teachings of *taiji* and their profound laws and principles in this book. I, like all other readers, have benefited mightily.

*Year of the heavenly stem gui and the earthly branch si, early winter*

---

Yu Hongkun began his training as a boy, learning the arts of grappling, striking, and long fist with his father. He formally joined the school of the renowned martial artist Lu Wenrui in order to study the methods of South Pole lineage white monkey *tongbiquan*.[6] At this time, he also became a formal disciple of Professor Ma Xianda in the study of the combat arts of *tongbei*,[7] which comprise the eight great opening methods, the eight great beckoning methods, the twelve great chopping fist gates, the twelve striking hands, the eight flashing turns, the stabbing kicks, and

---

[6] *Tongbiquan* is written "通臂拳."

[7] *Tongbei[quan]* is written "通背拳."

the nine-character praying mantis fists of *bajiquan*.⁸ Later, he earned the fondness of the famous modern-day *dachengquan* master and martial arts researcher Wang Xuanjie,⁹ who passed his lineage down to Yu Hongkun. After Master Wang Xuanjie bestowed with him a laudatory calligraphic scroll reading "Number one intercepting hand in *dachengquan*," Yu continued his studies with *dachengquan* master Chang Zhilang, thereby gaining a thorough understanding of this martial art's theories and combat applications. He is especially skilled in using weapons and in grappling.

Master Yu's books include *The Noble Truths of the Study of Dachengquan* (1997), a three-volume tome entitled *Dachengquan* (2001), *The Study of Dachengquan*, and *Selections on Studying and Imparting Dachengchuan*.

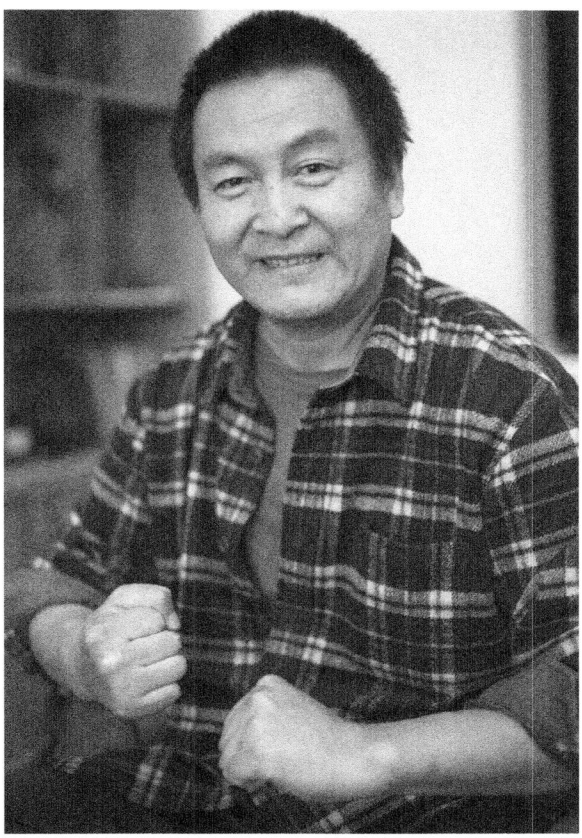

Master Yu Hongkun

---

⁸ The characters for *bajiquan* are "八極拳."

⁹ *Dachengquan* (大成拳) is another name for *yiquan* (意拳).

# Destined for *Taijiquan*

## *Author's Preface*

As a child I had the sort of constitution that people in Shanghai used to call "a herbal medicine pot." As early as I can remember, visits to the doctor were such a regular undertaking that if I was able to make it a whole two weeks without having to go to the hospital, the level of excitement at home would make you think somebody had announced a wedding. My parents and elders fretted constantly over my health, holding onto the hope of finding some trick or other that would strengthen my body and let me grow up without any setbacks.

Luckily, in spite of my early feebleness, I really liked martial arts. I idolized the warriors and masters in Chinese lore, and I yearned to answer the call of the fabled world of wandering, free-spirited fighters. I don't know if it was the heavens looking out for me, or my own good fortune or good karma, but somehow as a sickly, martial arts-loving boy I ended up having a neighbor named Wang Jurong, who was the daughter of Master Wang Ziping, the original head of the Shaolin department in the Central Guoshu Institute. Thanks to this happy coincidence, when I was about seven or eight years old, I began learning to how throw kicks and punches behind the adults as they practiced under Master Wang near my home. I trained more diligently than most other children my age, and as a result my health improved considerably, but even so my constitution remained so weak that it kept me from developing real martial skill. As a result of my lack of progress, I started to feel a bit ambivalent about the martial arts that I initially believed to be almost magical, but finding health after being a boy who was "so weak he couldn't even stand up to the wind" planted the seeds of a lifelong interest.

Some years later, on a Sunday morning when I was in high school, I had an unexpected encounter with a little old man in Fuxing Park in Shanghai that led me to fundamentally reassess everything I thought I knew about martial arts. The first time I saw this "little old man," Dong Bin, demonstrate the internal martial arts, I was simply dumbstruck—I felt like I was seeing something from another world. What struck me as especially remarkable was that this master, standing right before me doing things that seemed to belong in another realm, was actually extremely affable and approachable. My early childhood dreams were instantly rekindled, and I couldn't help but ask myself, "Is this the master I used to dream of finding when I was a sickly little boy?"

From that moment onwards, the first thought in my mind every Sunday morning was to go to the park to watch Dong Bin teach and train. But good things only come to those who wait, and it was only several years later, in 1987, when I formally bowed into Master Dong's lineage. It was then that my journey in search of the truth of *taiji* really began.

Dong Bin received his *taiji* knowledge via the transmissions of Master Yue Huanzhi[10] and Master Dong Shizuo, my two grand-teachers. Yue Huanzhi and Dong Shizuo were both *taiji* masters who enjoyed great fame in their times. In terms of forms, push hands, as well as actual combat, they were the types of martial sages who only pop up a few times each century. This was especially the case with my grand-teacher, Yue Huanzhi, who in addition to being incredibly achieved in the study of martial arts, was also a professor

---

[10] Master Ren's grand-teacher's surname (樂) is pronounced Yue, but there is another surname in China with the exact same character but a different pronunciation, "Le." For this reason, there are a number of texts in English that refer to Master Yue as "Le Huanzhi," and in fact some native Mandarin speakers who only know of Master Yue through the written record also pronounce his surname as Le.

at Zhendan University.[11] He wasn't merely an accomplished academic, but also highly regarded in Buddhist circles for being thoroughly versed in the sutras. In fact, Master Yue was the type of polymath who could deliver teachings from the three schools of Confucianism, Buddhism, and Daoism, finding the common threads linking all three traditions. While any scholar who is fully conversant in "the three teachings" would be considered a rarity, Master Yue took his erudition a step further, as he was able to clearly explain and plainly demonstrate the essence of internal martial arts using traditional Chinese and Buddhist philosophy. Master Yue enriched his predecessors' teachings by applying the wisdom of Confucianism and Buddhism to the worlds of internal martial arts and *taijiquan*, and as a result he elevated the techniques of *taijiquan* to a new level. One gets an inkling of Master Yue's skill and fame from the fact that, in his day, famous gentlemen of politics and commerce in Beijing and Shanghai considered it an honor just to have the chance to meet him. In the course of these behind-the-scenes meetings, Master Yue left behind numerous legends of fantastic skill, stories that are still told with great relish to this day in martial arts society.

I can only chalk it up to the grace of the heavens that Master Dong Bin, who had received such excellent *taijiquan* instruction from Yue Huanzhi and Dong Shizuo, decided to teach the young and still somewhat sickly me without the slightest reservation. He unlocked a treasure chest for me, transmitting insights into the truths of *taiji* that took him an entire lifetime to garner. Under my teacher's careful tutelage—as well as the watchful eyes of senior students like Guo Dadong—I made quick strides towards the inner sanctum of *taijiquan*'s mysteries, experiencing the unfolding of all manner of marvels both in my body and my spirit.

Following my initiation, I gradually learned to move my body and mind as one. My physique transformed to the degree that I became able to put the pearls of *taijiquan*'s essential teachings into practice no matter where I was and what I was doing. Over the course of decades

---

[11] 震旦大學.

of engaging with the subtleties of *taijiquan*'s methods, I came to realize that the wonders of Chinese culture simply cannot be appreciated by just hearing people talk about them. Rather, the marrow from each of the disciplines in traditional Chinese culture must be extracted through actual practice; an unwavering commitment to training must exist so that the teachings can be used for long-term self-cultivation. Practice and philosophy have a reciprocal relationship, and thus, on those days when a practitioner realizes something wondrous, he or she reaps the benefits both spiritually and physically. This is what allows a *taijiquan* student to learn to let movement and transformation flow directly from the mind. Whenever I have shared this opinion with masters in the older generations of martial artists, they have nodded with approval.

The principles of *taijiquan* derive from knowledge of the profound ways in which *yin* and *yang* harmoniously combine. The employment of these principles in combat is called "mysterious technique." When used to nurture good health, these principles can bring great benefits to the hearts and minds of everyday people, which is a much better way to put Chinese culture into practice than fighting!

When we turn our gazes upon modern society, we see that *taiji* training is moving further and further away from its nuclear principles. Some practitioners use the art's name, but don't comprehend its physical requirements; others understand how *taijiquan* is physically trained, but fail to blend its mind methods into their practice. Both ways are fruitless, and yet these degenerated practices have spread far and wide. Students of *taiji* like myself look upon this situation with lament, and we worry that we're not living up to our predecessors' wisdom, much less their painstaking efforts in creating this art.

I am no adept, and I still feel that I'm far from reaching a final understanding of the essence of *taijiquan*, but with the repeated encouragement of my elders and good friends, and after my own thorough consideration, I decided it would not be right to keep my insights to myself. Thus, I wrote this book in order to share my experiences from years of *taiji* practice, as well as to explain the core details of everything that was transmitted to me in my teacher's lineage. My hope is that those who share my interests will use this book as a reference, and that it will help them to one day enter into the proverbial inner court of *taijiquan*. In this way, I will fulfill a vow I made long ago, when I was praying before a statue of the Buddha to ask for inspiration: "Once I understand the art of *taijiquan*, if there are any others in the world with sincerity in their hearts who wish to understand this path, I will pour out the contents of my knowledge before them, holding absolutely nothing back!"

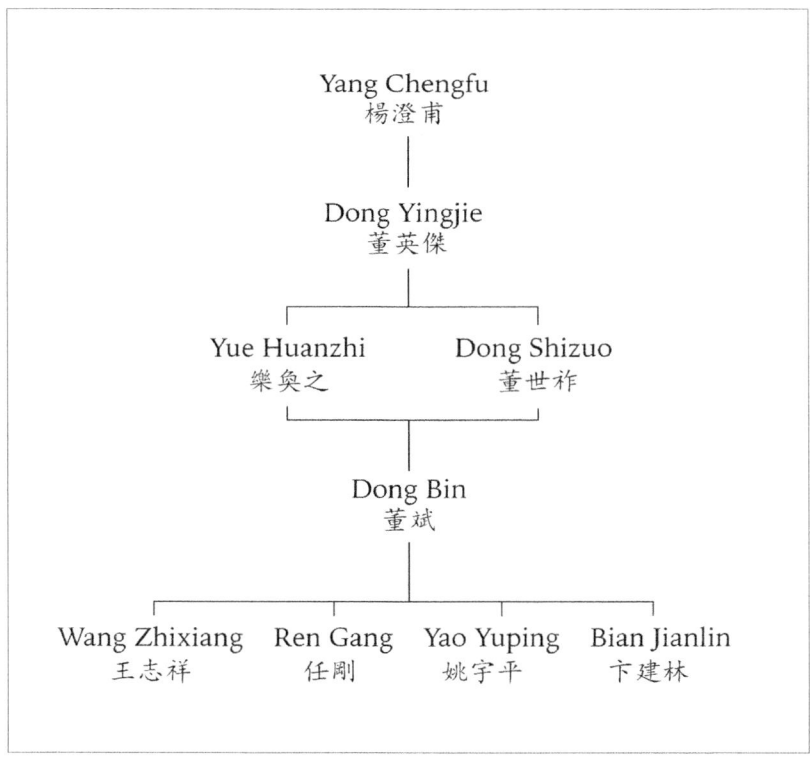

Dong Bin's lineage in Shanghai

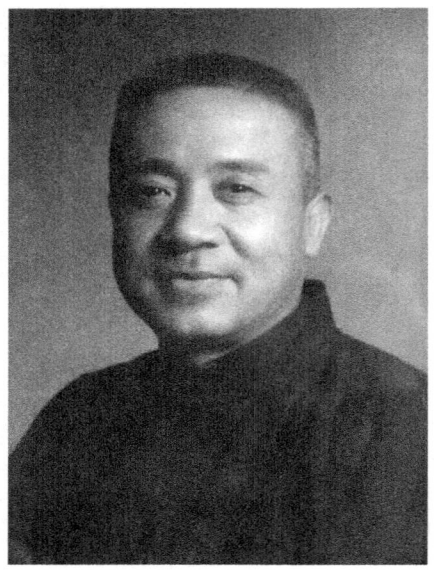

Master Yue Huanzhi

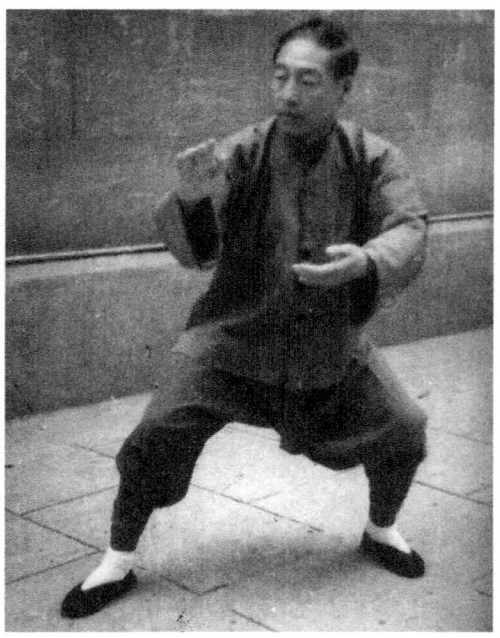

Master Dong Shizuo

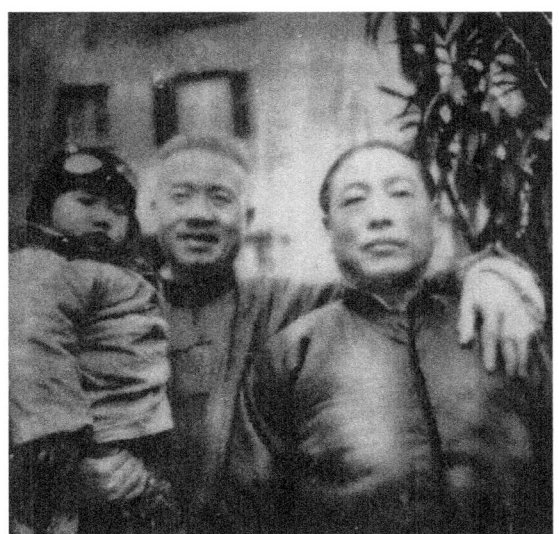

Yue Huanzhi and Dong Shizuo

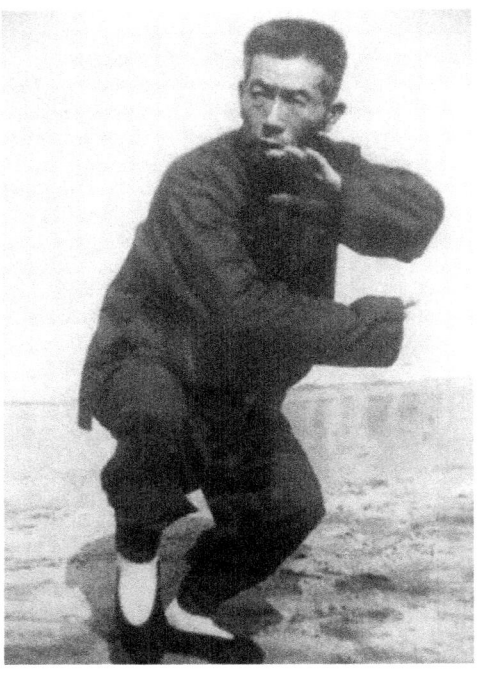

Master Dong Bin

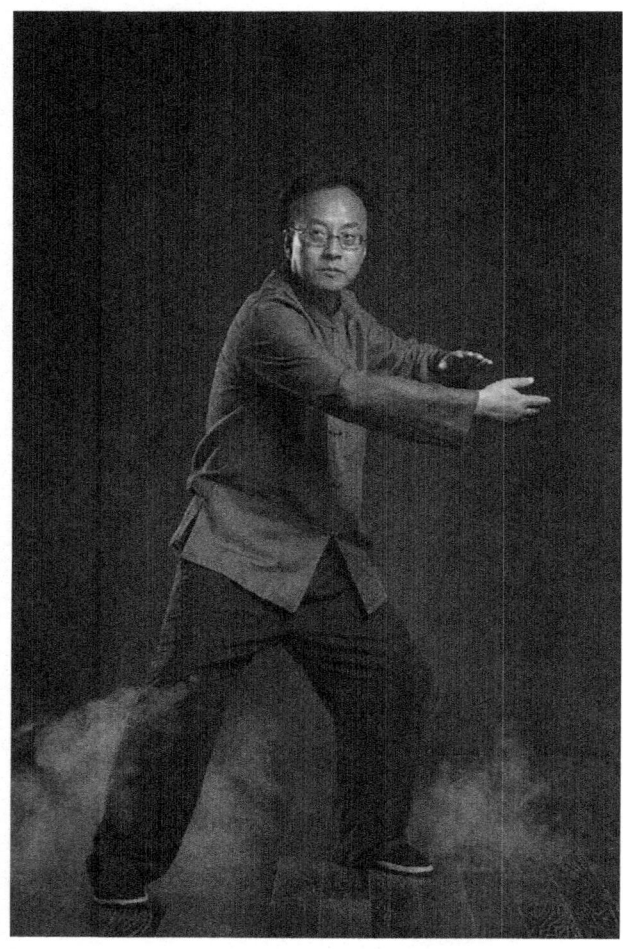

Ren Gang

# Notes on the English Edition

## *Translator's Introduction*

I FIRST MET Ren Gang in the spring of 2011, when his disciple and good friend of mine, Zhong Yingyang, invited me to join them for an outdoor lunch in an orchard in suburban Shanghai, where the peach trees were in full bloom. Yingyang had already spoken to me of the long, circuitous route he took before arriving at Ren's doorstep, and of the massive gulf between the "real" *taijiquan* Master Ren practices and teaches, and that which most other teachers are capable of presenting. At the time I still lacked the experience necessary to judge the merits of Yingyang's opinions, and not having had the chance to touch hands with Ren during the lunch, I found it difficult to believe that this fellow with a something of a polished gentleman's air knew much about the fighting arts.

Later that year, Yingyang invited me to attend a lecture Master Ren delivered at the Natural Path Academy in eastern Shanghai. Ren shared stories about his and some of his teachers' and grand-teachers' paths, and a whole lot of philosophical ideas tied to Daoism and Buddhism. I enjoyed the storytelling and philosophizing, but Master Ren did not demonstrate his martial skills during the event, and I walked away convinced that he was propounding theories of little practical value. Nevertheless, I couldn't write Ren off. At the time I was training Wudang martial arts under Master Gao Tieniao in People's Park, and it so happened that a fellow student, Chen Peng, knew Ren Gang and had also personally studied under Ren's teacher, the late Dong Bin. In addition to being able to perform martial arts forms with enviable grace, Chen Peng once gently twisted my wrist and made it almost impossible for me to move, even though I was not in any pain. After this, we got to talking about Dong Bin and Ren Gang. Chen Peng agreed that he found Ren's theories nearly incomprehensible, and said he figured that most of Ren's students were in the same boat. But, he said, while Ren's words may be difficult to fathom, whatever he is doing is most definitely real. Chen Peng enjoined me to never to pass up the chance to touch hands with Master Ren should one arise. As it happens, some years later he formally became Ren's disciple.

In 2013 I left Shanghai and returned to Beijing, nearly precluding any chance of finding my way to Ren Gang's studio. In 2017 I returned to the US for six months, more or less convinced I had reached an impassable plateau in my internal martial arts training. I had by then failed to meet a teacher who could or would demonstrate to me the kind of skill described in Wang Zongyue's *Treatise on Taijiquan*, and yet I was content to be thankful for what I had learned, and to simply keep practicing the things which clearly benefited my health. During this six month period, a good friend and fellow alumnus of the Beijing University of Chinese Medicine, Jeff Chen, was living nearby in rural Connecticut. Since he had reached a similar plateau on his own path in martial arts, we began meeting once a week to train for as long as ten hours at a time. We put down almost all of the forms and techniques either of us had learned in our combined four decades of training, and instead began exploring internal martial arts principles in a completely pared-down manner.

To our shock, by removing everything but the fundamental points of *taiji* philosophy and the simple act of pushing on another human being, we began to be able to do things that seemed impossible. As the months wore on and our experience deepened, we became capable of dispatching with quite aggressive, full-strength attacks from one another by keeping the mind and the body empty. While ours was a controlled training environment and we were under no illusion that we could maintain the empty state in an unexpected brawl or in an MMA ring, we could see that we had at long last tapped into something that was more than mere imagination. And, to my further surprise, the language that we used to communicate our insights to one another began to sound more and more like the contents of the lecture I heard Ren Gang deliver in Shanghai six years prior.

I began digging up bits and pieces of Ren's writings online, and it was clear that his words had simply flown over my head when I first heard them. Coincidentally, in 2016 Zhong Yingyang had asked me if I would be willing to translate Ren's book. I sent him an email in the spring of 2018 to ask if Ren was still hoping to put out an English version, and Yingyang replied that he was. I was by then living in Taiwan, but I made a point of scheduling a stopover in Shanghai during my next work trip to China. On my first visit, Ren still gave off his trademark coiffed, vaguely aristocratic air, but I was no longer looking for the blatant signs of martial prowess an actor in the role of a kung-fu master might be expected to exude. After satisfying himself that my linguistic abilities were up to the task of rendering his book in English, Ren stood up and suggested we touch hands, to make sure I would get a *feel* for things that defy conveyance through words. As I document in detail in the many footnotes in this book drawn from sparring with Ren Gang, it was anything but a disappointing experience. I was terribly outmatched, not because of Ren's size or strength or speed, but because of something else altogether. That *something else*, it is our hope, is pointed to as clearly as can be between the two covers of this book. To taste that something else, is to taste *taiji*.

## How to Read This Book

*The Heart Treasure of Taijiquan* is based on 《太極拳行法釋要》 (*Tai Ji Quan Xing Fa Shi Yao*), which was published by the Shanghai Lexicographical Publishing House in 2013. The book comprises a mix of essays, exegeses, lecture transcripts, and answers to questions put to Ren by his students and readers. Being essentially a compilation, this work lacks the structure typical of books that were written as a single manuscript. Nevertheless, having likely read the book more times than anybody else on the planet, I feel that there is a certain logic to the order in which the materials are presented, and I strongly suggest that readers work through the chapters in order. Of course, there's nothing wrong with jumping ahead to read Ren's commentary on "The Cat's Marvelous Methods." But to any reader who does so, I suggest reading it a second time later on, after going back to the beginning to digest the preceding chapters. Ren's exegesis of the old story of the cat will yield much deeper meaning to a person who is already familiar with his core *taijiquan* teachings.

In almost all instances in this book, I have transliterated terms using *Hanyu pinyin*, which was developed in the People's Republic of China and has become the worldwide standard for Romanizing modern Mandarin. However, Chinese characters appear in their traditional forms, which remain in official use in the city of Hong Kong and the nation of Taiwan. I opted to use traditional characters because they are the basis for research into ancient writings, as well as for connecting to the classical aspects of Chinese culture that the communist party has worked so violently to disrupt. The simplification of Chinese characters was a solution to illiteracy in the era of handwriting. In the age of typing on computers and phones, simplified Chinese characters—which were often stripped of both meaning and beauty—are obsolete, and their continued usage has more to do with their role in totalitarian "newspeak" than anything else.

Footnotes explaining the specialized vocabulary of *taijiquan* that Ren uses appear throughout the book. Whenever possible, I used English terms instead of *pinyin*, and in each instance when I had to choose a word for a complicated concept, I made sure to ask Master Ren to provide me detailed explanations and demonstrations during our in-person meetings. I took notes during those meetings which then became footnotes that inform the reader precisely what Ren intended to express with the vocabulary he uses. Please note that some of Master Ren's interpretations of common *taijiquan* terminology may be quite different from other teachers' or authors'. Please also note that footnotes only accompany a new term the first time it appears, so skipping ahead in the text may mean becoming confused by the appearance of arcane-seeming terms that were already glossed elsewhere.

Finally, bilingual readers will notice that I made changes to the original which can only be called "editorial." The simplest changes involved breaking up extremely long sentences and paragraphs. I also frequently had to slightly change the order of sentences within a paragraph, eliminate redundancies, and generally do my best to increase readability instead of producing a pedantically faithful translation. I made these changes with Master Ren's support and guidance, as well as the strong encouragement of his good friend and original choice for translating his book, the pianist Paul Leu.

## How to Use This Book

Being its translator has forced me to read Ren Gang's book over and over again throughout the course of the last two years. Returning to it every few months, while keeping up with my own not-especially-rigorous training regimen, has made each new visit to the text a source of surprising insights that tangibly improve my practice.[12] More times than I can count, when I return after a year to a portion of the text that left little impression on me when I first I read or translated it, I suddenly find previously-unseen gems of knowledge glittering on the page. When the time is ripe to encounter them, this book's teachings are always easy to apply, and the kinds of results they yield are as profound as Ren promises. But had I not experimented with Ren's teachings in the months between readings, the import of statements I overlooked the first few times I read them would never have become apparent. This book is full of treasures, but they cannot all be unearthed in a single reading, and most of them will be useless to those who don't train.

---

[12] For curious readers I should add that I never had the time to learn the eighty-eight move *taijiquan* form that Ren Gang teaches. Instead, I adopted the standing practice he taught me (the instructions he gave me in person are no different from what is presented in this book) and integrated his teachings on the lumbar and *mingmen* as well as "equipollence" with the *xingyiquan* and *baguazhang* movements I had already learned elsewhere.

Beyond pointing out the benefit of reading this book more than once, I am reluctant to try to tell readers how to experiment with Master Ren's instructions. I can say with confidence that Ren Gang made these teachings accessible to the public in book form with the hope that readers will find a way to integrate them with their practices of *taijiquan* and other martial arts (as well as life in general). On the other hand, he stresses several times in this book that having an in-person teacher is still a necessity. This could present a conundrum, as surely few *taijiquan* teachers in the world today teach as Ren does. Nevertheless, as one of my Daoist teachers has reminded me countless times over the years, it is the nature of the Dao to resolve all contradictions. Readers with a deep affinity for the wisdom contained in these pages will undoubtedly find a way to experience it directly.

The English title of this book is an homage to *The Heart Treasure of the Enlightened Ones*, a commentary on the 19th century Tibetan Buddhist master Patrul Rinpoche's teachings, written by the great 20th century master Dilgo Khyentse Rinpoche, who was one of the fourteenth Dalai Lama's primary teachers. While I daren't place this book's contents on the same pedestal as those two important lamas' teachings (nor, I think, would Master Ren), the title choice was not a flippant one. For starters, this book's Chinese title is itself an homage to the title of a commentary on the *Shurangama Sutra* dear to Ren Gang's heart. Additionally, just as *The Heart Treasure of the Enlightened Ones* contains a modern master's exegesis of a piece of writing created during the tail end of the pre-modern era in Tibet, this work contains Ren's explications of Wang Zongyue's *Treatise on Taijiquan*, a piece of writing dating to China's Ming dynasty. Furthermore, even though it is necessary to seek out living teachers to truly learn Buddhism, books like *The Heart Treasure of the Enlightened Ones* can serve as tremendously important sources of inspiration and clarification for Buddhist practitioners. Similarly, committed students of *taijiquan* may find that this book serves to inspire and clarify, hopefully filling in blanks and perhaps opening up new gateways on a path that must also include training under a teacher's careful guidance. Finally, there is a strong connection between Master Ren's lineage and Tibetan Buddhism. According to Ren, Master Yue Huanzhi only achieved mastery of *taijiquan* after commencing to study and practice Tibetan Buddhism. Ren Gang himself attributes his own success in entering into *taijiquan*'s mysteries to the consequences of a vow he made before a statue of the Buddha in a temple in Shanghai—it is because of that vow that *The Heart Treasure of Taijiquan* now exists. Such a strong connection between the ostensibly Daoist art of *taijiquan* and Vajrayana Buddhism may seem odd to some. And yet, those who pay close attention to Tibetan Buddhist *thangka* paintings will notice that the *taiji* symbol and the eight trigrams appear on them quite frequently. There has in fact been dialogue between Daoism and Tibetan Buddhism since at least the Tang dynasty.

## Translator's Acknowledgements

I offer my thanks to Ren Gang for entrusting me with this project, and for sharing with me in person the fruits of his lifelong devotion to Chinese martial arts, philosophy, and self-cultivation. I also thank Zhong Yingyang for playing a pivotal role in getting this project off of the ground.

I am extremely grateful to all of my own teachers and mentors in the Chinese martial arts and self-cultivation traditions. In the order in which I met them they are: Master Kwan Cortez, Sifu Antoine Wiley, Peter Moy, Master Raymond Ly, Dr. Peter Caughey, Wen Su, Master Cheng Aiping, Teacher Luo at White Cloud Monastery, Ven. Meng-Can, Master Gao Tieniao, Dr. Wu Guozhong, Abbess Liu Yuanhui, Master Liu Xuyang, Dr. Andrew Nugent-Head, and Professor Liu Tsung-Min. I also offer the deepest gratitude to my mother, father, and brothers: Lina, Peter, Samuel, and Juan Diego. Finally, deep thanks are owed to those who have supported my studies, including Ven. Chien-Ch'ing, Mr. Lin Chaoxiang, the Ministry of Education of Taiwan, and the Office of International Affairs at National Taiwan University.

I thank Ryan Crocombe, William Su, and Jonah Katz for going through drafts of this translation with fine-toothed combs and offering valuable advice. Special thanks are owed to the late Michael Becker, who made numerous suggestions after reading an early draft, contributed to this project in other ways, and began encouraging me to do work like this back in 2013—it was an honor knowing you, brother. I also thank Liang Dehua, Benoit Amoyel, and Mark Parzynski for kindly helping the publisher and I find the photographs of Yang Chengfu that appear in this book, despite our never having met. Anne-Maree Taranto and Barbara Tada have my gratitude for their excellent design work. Last but not least, I tip my hat to Johan Hausen at the Purple Cloud Institute for patiently keeping this project moving along and offering plenty of assistance and advice, as well as to Daniel Spigelman for opening the door.

I dedicate the labors of this work of translation to two movements that inspired and humbled me during its undertaking. My work on this project began in earnest in the summer of 2019, when people of all ages in Hong Kong shocked the world by standing up by the millions to demand the human rights, civil rights, democracy, freedom, and self-determination that I have taken for granted my entire life, except for during the ten years that I lived in the cynically-named "people's republic" of China. I drafted this introduction in June of 2020, as the United States was snapped awake by protests sparked by the murders of Ahmaud Arbery, Breonna Taylor, and George Floyd, three names on an endless list of Americans deprived of the most fundamental of supposedly-inalienable rights so that a racist caste system may prolong its brutal existence. Working safely behind my laptop, far from the physical and bureaucratic weaponry aimed at the protestors in Hong Kong and the US—not to mention the inmates of the carceral behemoths befouling both nations—I am reminded constantly that what rights any of us enjoy are precious, precarious, incomplete, and far-too-unevenly distributed. To all people standing up against injustice and oppression in all lands, I bow humbly and gratefully. May you brave ones taking stands for justice each find *taiji*, and in so doing may you find inexhaustible wells of inner peace, clarity, and strength to draw upon as you push hands with the will to tyranny, wherever it is found, without and within.

Last but neva least: Shout out to the Lizards Crew Nation, 825, The Industry Shakedown on WHPK, and the whole NSN squad. And like the man Rebel said: Kiser Lived… *Did You?*

*Mattias Daly/慈明修*
*Taipei, in the 109th year of the R.O.C.*

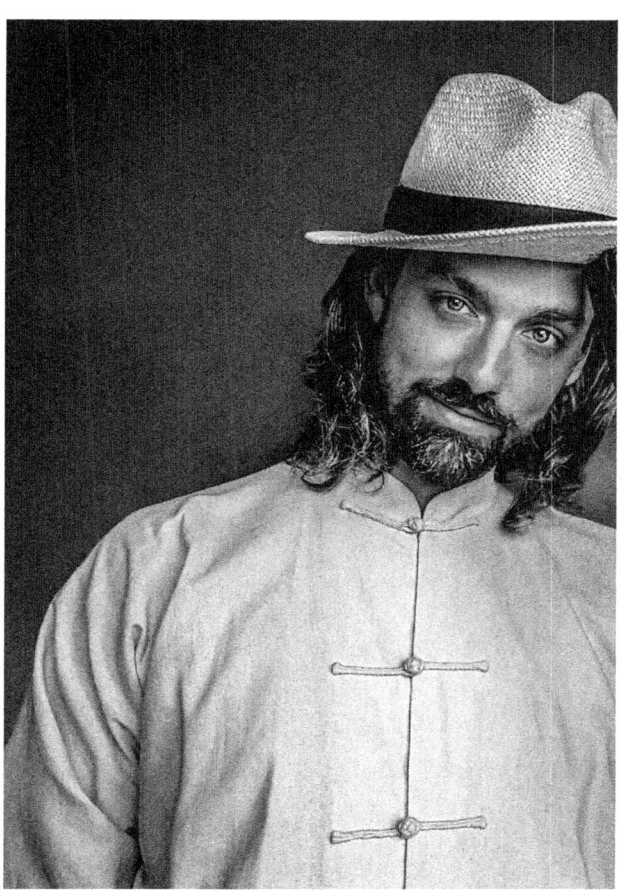

Mattias Daly (Photo: Steve Yu/Syphargenic)

# 1

## On Culture

*Putting Chinese culture into practice via* taijiquan

MOST PEOPLE PRACTICE *taijiquan* for one of two reasons. The first reason stems from dreams of becoming a warrior—the person who is thusly motivated hopes that through *taijiquan* practice he or she will become a formidable member of the martial arts world. A lot of young *taiji* students have dreams like this. The second reason usually appears after a person has reached middle age and established a successful career, when suddenly the person discovers he or she has exchanged health for worldly success. After long years with their shoulder to the wheel, people often wish to do something that nourishes life. Naturally, *taijiquan* is a good choice.

There is, however, a third reason for practicing *taijiquan*. It is one that gets overlooked, and yet it just so happens to be where the soul of *taijiquan* is found. When training for this reason, one uses *taijiquan* to put the philosophical teachings of Chinese culture into actual practice. Absent this goal, *taijiquan* risks becoming nothing more than a set of movements that are not necessarily any better than any other type of physical exercise.

In the classical Chinese sense, one is only cultured if one's learning is embodied in skill—not simply in ideas and knowledge—and *taijiquan* practice can be a way to achieve such embodiment. These days a lot of people are studying aspects of traditional Chinese culture. Some study Buddhism or Daoism, perhaps by reading Buddhist sutras or reading the *Daodejing*. Others study Confucian texts such as *The Analects, The Great Learning,* and so forth. But only a small minority of students manage to take what they have studied and apply it in ways that allow them to alter their characters and their behavior. The problem is not that the ancient sages' words were useless. Rather, the problem is that many people mistakenly conclude that the sages were no more than theorists, and that their teachings are little more than stimulating topics for dinner table conversation. When this happens we get little real help from our studies, and learning how to cultivate our bodies and nourish our essential natures is out of the question.

Becoming authentically cultured in the classical Chinese sense is something that is brought about through real practice. Academic knowledge is no substitute for real practice. That Laozi, Confucius, and other sages were able to move the masses and change people—that they were able to "manage their families, govern their nations, and create peace on earth,"[13] as one famous Confucian maxim puts it—was due to their actual life skill, not to tongue wagging. Therefore, if one wishes to properly study Chinese culture, one must begin with practice. Only after we develop skill in restoring our bodies and nourishing our mind natures do we begin to glimpse the path walked by the great, virtuous sages of the past. *Taijiquan* so happens to be one of the best gates through which to embark upon this journey.

If one wishes to experience the true meaning of *taijiquan* and have it become a vehicle for putting Chinese culture into practice, then one must begin with its principles. The old Yang family writings said, "If one grasps the principle that heaven and earth are of one body, then naturally one gains the primordial *qi* that flows from the sun and moon." The principle that heaven and earth are of one body is the foundation of *taiji*. This foundation is called *"wuji."*[14]

---

[13] This well-known phrase, abbreviated from *The Great Learning* (《大學》), reads "齊家，治國，平天下." Ren examines it shortly.

[14] The characters for *wuji* are "無極."

The ancients used a "◯" to represent the principle of an individual human merged with all things. This concept implies that self, others, the heavens, and the earth are all within the range of one's own perception. In modern terms, this range is what we often refer to as our "*qi* field." The classic *The Great Learning* discusses considerations key to Confucian ways of cultivating one's person and nourishing original nature. It instructs readers to "examine phenomena to obtain wisdom."[15] "Examine phenomena" is not an instruction to go off and conduct research into all things in creation, nor is it an instruction for you to rule out your material desires. Rather, it suggests that we observe the myriad things with our senses and thereby achieve a state of mind that allows us to perceive all things. Such a state is synonymous with what Daoism calls *wuji*. This task is foundational to internal martial arts because force is produced by the movements of *qi* fields.

The next sentence in *The Great Learning* teaches, "Let your thinking be sincere to rectify your heart."[16] This line tells us to employ our capability to sense and perceive the myriad things as we interact with all the objects and phenomena we encounter, and then, having received feedback from all things and phenomena, to cultivate right intentions and behaviors. This process does not need to be contrived; a person who possesses excellent powers of perception will naturally be disinclined to doing negative deeds. That is why Mencius said, "People of noble character thus avoid the slaughterhouse." He meant that keen perception makes it hard for a person to gaze with indifference at others in pain.[17]

The process Confucians call "making your thoughts sincere and rightening your heart" dovetails with the process of "cultivating

---

[15] The passage Ren mentions here is commonly abbreviated as a *chengyu*, "格物致知."

[16] This passage is commonly abbreviated as the *chengyu* "正心誠意."

[17] Mencius' original words were "是以君子遠庖廚也."

your person."[18] In *taijiquan*, this means the process of refining *jing* to transform it into primordial *qi*.[19] This process involves converting later heaven *jing* and *qi* into a prior heaven *wuji* energy field.[20] Once

---

[18] This term, "修身," appears in *The Great Learning* as the prerequisite to "managing one's household, governing the nation, and creating peace on earth." It follows upon "making thoughts sincere to rectify the heart." Self, character, and the body are all implied by "身," which I translate here as "person," following James Legge.

[19] *Jing* is from "精," a term discussed in depth in any introductory text for Chinese medicine or Daoist inner alchemy. Broadly, it refers to the physical (as opposed to energetic and psychic) constituents of the human body. More narrowly, it can refer to all manner of bodily fluids, and the body's ability to produce them in healthy quality and quantity. Even more narrowly, it can refer to sexual fluids, especially semen, as well as the "life force" that is implied by their role in reproduction. Finally, in Daoist alchemical texts based upon the eight trigrams, the word *jing* may be used symbolically to refer to primordial *jing* and *qi* or even primordial *shen*, while in Laozi's *Daodejing* its meaning can be yet more abstruse. In light of the above, readers should be careful not to treat *jing* and semen as simple synonyms.

Primordial *qi* is from "元氣." Ren here uses this term as a synonym for *Qi* or 炁, which is introduced in chapter two and discussed many times throughout the book.

[20] This term comes from the characters "先天," which literally means "prior [to] heaven," but could be more thoroughly translated as "that which is precedes the genesis of the cosmos," or more simply as "prenatal." It refers to the unmanifest, realmless realm that is beyond duality. Being beyond duality, it is beyond any conceptual notions of existence and of non-existence. Being unlimited by distinctions between existence and non-existence, it is also unlimited by concepts and senses of time. Therefore, while we may say that this term points to something "prior" to the manifest universe, we must know that it is not a concept to which temporal distinctions apply. For that reason, although the prior heaven state came "before" everything we know, it is also eternally present and accessible. Daoist practice, with its emphases on "non-doing" and "not knowing," leads in this apparently paradoxical direction.

The opposite of prior heaven, "later heaven," is written as "後天." It refers to the realm of manifest existence where all things are defined by duality. The first character can also be understood to mean "after," whereas the second character—literally meaning "heavens" or "cosmos"—may be understood as representing the genesis of all that exists, commonly called "the ten thousand things" in classical Daoist writings. Thus, inasmuch as it

you have cultivated your perceptive powers, your concomitantly increasing strength will become as though infectious, and you will begin to transform the people around you. This is what is implied in the next instruction in *The Great Learning*, "manage your family," which in *taijiquan* is the process of refining *qi* to transform it into *shen*. If you have vast *qi* that fills everything between heaven and earth and transforms your fellow countrymen and women, then, as *The Great Learning* says, you can "govern the nation." Finally, if you become like Confucius, a person whose strength continues to transform others centuries after his passing, then you can "create peace on earth."

In sum, the arc of training in *taijiquan* is a process of putting Confucianism and Daoism into practice. This means it's a process of truly restoring your body and nourishing your original nature. It is in these transformations where the ultimate meaning of *taijiquan* lies. If you reject these ideas, then if you're a martial artist you would probably be better off just training in external martial arts, grappling, or boxing. It doesn't matter how beautiful your movements are or how particular you are about training—if you train *taijiquan* without attending to these principles, then your practice has nothing to do with real *taiji*. Even its health-promoting effects won't necessarily be better than those you would create with any other sort of exercise.

## Do you treat your culture like a son, or like a pig?

Recently I got together with some friends in Sanlin District in Shanghai. After dinner we went for a stroll in the old town before settling down in a tea house to sample their finest offerings while we chatted. Next to the tea house was a martial arts academy, and upon asking we discovered that some Chen style *taijiquan* teachers had just incorporated a new company and were preparing to open for business. It so happened that the marketing coordinator for the company, a

---

can refer to the birth of all things, "postnatal" is sometimes used to translate this term.

gentleman from Hong Kong, was in the tea house with us. My friends and I, all of us being infatuated with martial arts, invited him to join us for tea.

This fellow was extremely loquacious, and he bubbled with enthusiasm as he outlined his marketing strategy. After hearing him out I was quite shocked—it turned out this gentleman didn't know the first thing about Chinese *taiji* culture or martial arts, but he was overflowing with confidence in his eyebrow-raising scheme. The company's goal was to open a large number of training centers before the famous elderly Chen style *taijiquan* master affiliated with the company passed away. While the esteemed old master remained alive, they would spare no expense attracting people to join these centers. In order to hook new students, they redesigned the traditional Chen style *taijiquan* forms in line with the notion that the *"yin"* and *"yang"* of *taiji* philosophy are references to males and females, and declared that men should push hands with women so that *"yin* and *yang* can nourish one another."  Another of their measures was to employ hunky men and pretty women as coaches.

I was alarmed by what I heard. I responded to the marketing director, "When you do things this way, the result is that these people will never be able to experience real *taiji*—what will become of the culture in the long run?" He bluntly replied that his company's train of thought is more suited to the needs of the majority than the old ways are, and that the business would find success by being a platform for finding dates. I sighed and remarked that he didn't understand *taiji*, and then proceeded to explain its philosophical background to him. To my surprise he paid rapt attention, and then followed up with a long stream of questions. Finally, noticing that the hour had drawn late, I said to him, "I don't want to keep lecturing you, but I'm certain that if you had a better understanding of *taijiquan* you wouldn't have the heart to go on degrading it the way you are. Think about if it were your own son—from the moment he was born you'd be fostering his talents to help him become a useful person. Who thinks about making money off his son from the moment he's born?" Unbelievably, after hearing me out, the fellow gave a guffaw and replied, "You treat *taiji* like it's your son, I treat it like it's a pig. As long as I can unload it at the market today, then tomorrow it's got nothing to do with me. You think I'm trying to be in this silly business for the rest of my life?"

When I heard this I said that I was deeply offended. The fellow responded frankly, "But isn't this just the way all cultural businesses are nowadays?" Indeed, he had a point. The general picture of modern companies that claim to promote traditional Chinese culture is one in which profiteering comes before anything else. Their way of doing things may make it seem like our culture is bursting back to life, but if you take a long-term view you will see that their approach is exacting grievous harm on the culture. For example, companies offering classes in *taijiquan* or in classical Chinese philosophy attract people from all around the world who admire these famous products of Chinese civilization. But countless people come and study for a year or two only to conclude that they didn't learn anything of practical use—to say nothing of having wondrous epiphanies or being moved to the cores of their beings—and then naturally enough they return home full of contempt. If people who saw Chinese culture as profound and worthy of respect before starting to study it ultimately come to look down upon it and leave in disgust, then great damage is being done! Today's Chinese martial arts are seen as flowery performance pieces, while today's traditional Chinese medicine is seen as pseudoscientific and superstitious. Ironically, these problems stem directly from the very people out there "promoting" the culture!

I believe that for people to properly promote this culture, they must first truly experience its essence, which means that their public endeavors must be founded in personal practice. Allowing the culture to shine by actually embodying it is more than enough to attract students who will wish to learn more. In fact, the precise thing diminishing traditional culture's lustre is all of the "promotion" going on. In the case of promoting *taijiquan*, the only thing a teacher needs to do is get each student to have experiences of using force, comprehending the principles of oneness, and feeling balance. Nobody who has tasted these things will fail to fall in love with this art.

There are two keys to furthering *taijiquan*'s development. The first is the fostering of inheritors. A number of promising young individuals with equal parts scholastic and martial talent must be nurtured, so that there will be a new generation of teachers who are capable of demonstrating the philosophical underpinnings of *taiji* in their martial artistry. The second key is the fostering of general hobbyists. Whenever hobbyists gain real insights into *taiji* philosophy by practicing *taijiquan*, they then joyously imbue their own areas of specialty with the epiphanies *taiji* practice has given them. An example of this is a French friend of mine, the pianist Paul Leu. His *taijiquan* training didn't turn him into a martial arts master, but even so he developed a *taiji*-based method of teaching piano, and now professional pianists frequently arrive at his doorstep to study with him. That is what "promoting" a culture really means! I'm sure insights from *taijiquan* could be used in golf or any other pursuit. When something is real, it attracts people simply by bringing them tangible benefits and enjoyment. The main challenge is that since real teachings don't yield instant returns, they tend not to be given a platform and they're often deprived of resources. This is a pity. If this deprivation is not rectified, the decline of our culture will only continue.

2

# ON TRAINING

*Prerequisite knowledge for successful* taijiquan *practice: On "qi" and "Qi"*

TAIJIQUAN HAS ENJOYED a recent surge in popularity. I've met business leaders, politicians, and movie stars who all say they love *taijiquan*. Meanwhile, a lot of people have devoted a lot of energy to promoting *taijiquan* and opening martial arts studios, but they generally present *taijiquan* as little more than another form of physical exercise. In modern *taiji* studios one frequently hears students asking things like, "Is my standing meditation posture very standard? Does doing it this way look any good?" Only rarely do people probe *taijiquan*'s depths and the philosophical background that led to its creation.

Anybody who wishes to discover the secrets contained within *taijiquan* must start by understanding the fundamental difference between the Chinese characters for *"qi"* and *"Qi."*[21] It has always

---

[21] The former character, transliterated in the lower case, is "氣." The latter, transliterated in the upper case, is "炁." Both are pronounced in the fourth tone in modern Mandarin. It should be noted that in countless classical and modern writings the character 氣 is used in ways that imply 炁. In such cases it is usually clear from context that something "prior heaven" is being discussed. An example of this potentially confusing phenomenon occurs momentarily, when Ren Gang references Mencius' idea of "vast, righteous *qi*," which actually pertains to *Qi*. Due to the inherent flexibility of the Chinese language, there are many other instances in this book where the character

been the case that most people practice *taijiquan* without reaching the levels of prior generations of masters, and this is often because they do not appreciate the distinction between "*qi*" and "*Qi*." The key to the gate to cultivating one's person and nourishing the mind's original nature is hidden in these two Chinese characters.

There are two prerequisites for developing skill in *taijiquan*. One is that a student must experience himself or herself, others, heaven, and earth as all being a single entity. The other is that a student must simultaneously encompass *yin* and *yang* within the scope of his or her perception. Before a student can wrap his or her mind around this very abstract-sounding problem, the distinction between "*qi*" and "*Qi*" must be clearly understood. In modern times both *qi* and *Qi* tend to be written with a single character—"氣"—but at a certain point in history only *qi* was written in this way, whereas *Qi* was written as "炁." In antiquity, *qi* and *Qi* were two wholly different concepts.

"氣" refers to what Daoism and Chinese medicine call "later heaven *qi*." After we eat, food's essences are transformed into our bodies' *qi* and blood, which were traditionally thought to be produced in the thoracic region, spleen, and stomach. In classical Chinese medicine, it is generally held that when there is insufficient *qi* and blood in the five *zang* organs of the human body, then the *qi* and blood of the kidneys are drawn upon to make up the difference; when there is a surplus of *qi* and blood in the five *zang* organs,[22] then it goes to the kidneys, which also replenish the *dantian*.[23] Being mostly a product of physical substances, later heaven *qi* can only help provide a foun-

---

氣 is used in a way that implies 炁, and as such "*qi*" and "*Qi*" both appear throughout the manuscript. As a rule of thumb, whenever Ren is discussing *taiji* philosophy or applications of *taijiquan*, he is referring to *Qi*, whereas *qi* is mostly used in health-related discussions. (O reader, I know how you feel—now you know where my grey hairs come from!)

[22] The character "臟" is generally rendered in *pinyin* in English writings on Chinese medicine as "*zang*." It refers to the organs understood to store the body's essences and spirits. They are the heart, liver, spleen, lungs, and kidneys.

[23] This *pinyin* word comes from the characters "丹田," literally "field of elixir." In this context, *dantian* refers to the place in the lower abdomen where *qi* can

dation for healthy cultivation practice; it is not directly related to cultivation itself.

"炁" is prior heaven *qi*, which is produced by the "refining of *jing* so that it turns into *Qi*." According to the ancients, when *jing* is turned into *qi* while one is in a state devoid of thought, the result is "*Qi*." Confucians call this "vast, righteous *qi*"[24] and Daoists also call it "*wuji*." This notion pertains to a field and to the power of consciousness within that field. It is not a substance inside of the human body. Rather, it represents the entirety of a person's scope of awareness. When this field—that is, the range of a practitioner's perception— comes under a person's powers of influence and command, then it is said that "*Qi* has transformed into *shen*." *Shen*, which is sometimes translated as "spirit," describes result of the transformation by which *Qi* becomes something that the practitioner is aware of and can use.

In terms of practice, the ability to maintain this state of awareness begins with the transformation of *jing* into *Qi*. As the aptitude of a student learning *taijiquan* gradually increases, his or her range of perception will effectively become his or her range of influence. *Qi* becomes *shen* as this range of influence transforms into a type of energy.

Some readers will be familiar with the oft-mentioned trinity of *jing*, *qi*, and *shen*,[25] but it is important to understand that *shen* is arrived at via *jing* and *Qi*. *Shen* is not intimately connected to *qi*. This is not to say that the later heaven *qi* associated with *qi* and blood has no

---

be stored, refined, and generated. This term does not refer to an anatomical organ; it relates to *qi* and *Qi*.

[24] From "浩然正氣." Ren argues that, strictly speaking, although the character 氣 is used here, the meaning of 炁 is implied.

[25] *Shen* is from "神." As with *jing* (and *qi*), its discussion is central to books on Chinese medicine and Daoist inner alchemy. Not directly translatable, *shen*'s implications include consciousness, mental activity, and mental energy, as well as what might be called "spirit" or "soul," if not "divine nature." *Jing*, *qi*, and *shen* are often discussed as a tripartite concept and sometimes called the "three treasures." The health of these three factors is closely interrelated in human life, and, as Ren reminds us, individual evolution can in many ways be seen as a question of refining *jing*, *qi*, *Qi*, and *shen*.

relationship whatsoever with *taijiquan*.[26] There is indeed a connection, because after blood has been nourished by *qi*, the five organs' healthy *qi* will assist in promoting the process of *Qi*'s transformation into *shen*. For instance, when our kidneys' later heaven *qi* is ample, it can do one of two things. The first is to transform into sexual fluids, which yearn to leave the body; the second is to transform into *jing*, which can then become *Qi*. If you undertake this process of conversion, then you're on the cultivator's path. *Taijiquan* is an uncanny process that allows us to move from the realm of *qi* to the realm of *Qi*. Once again, *Qi* is distinct from the *qi* from food that functions in our bodies. Understanding this point is extremely important!

When Sun Lutang met Song Shirong and asked him the difference between internal and external martial arts, Master Song replied, "Those who excel at nurturing *qi* are internalists, and those who don't excel at nurturing *qi* are externalists." With this simple answer, Song Shirong echoed Mencius' maxim, "nurture vast *qi*," thereby laying bare the mysteries of the internal martial arts for Sun Lutang.[27]

Sun Lutang did not yet understand, and in response to Song Shirong's answer he said that this must mean that an internalist is one whose *dantian* is full. Master Song corrected him forcefully, saying, "Wrong! Wrong! Although you have opened up the *qi* in your lower abdomen, if you don't transform it into power, then in the end it will inevitably harm you. Yours is not the highest path!" To thoroughly flesh out his philosophy, Song Shirong then added, "If you aren't enlightened to these tenets, then even if you train until you're as agile as a bird in flight or strong enough to lift eight tons, you'll be no more than an ordinary man with bestial strength, and you'll never move beyond the external arts." The great Sun Lutang was no different from anybody else. To develop a true understanding of

---

[26] In Chinese medicine, *qi* and blood are viewed as a single paired entity, with *qi* acting as blood's source of energy and life, and blood acting as *qi*'s material basis and source of sustenance. This *yin-yang* pair is very much a part of later heaven *qi*.

[27] Mencius said "我養吾浩然之氣." Both Mencius' and Song's quotes present tricky instances where the character 氣 is used to imply the character 炁.

Chinese culture and *taijiquan*, he had to begin by learning to distinguish *qi* and *Qi*.

## The three indispensable factors in taijiquan practice: A destination, a vessel, and a way to power your vessel

People frequently ask me, "Is that Yang family *taijiquan* that you're practicing? Or is it Chen family *taijiquan*? Which type of *taijiquan* is the best?" These questions reflect a lack of fundamental knowledge. *Taiji* is a philosophical foundation, while *taijiquan* is a method of combat that emerged from this foundation.[28] There is only one criterion for judging *taijiquan*: Is it executed by a practitioner who is in the *taiji* state, or not?

The amateurish questions above are akin to asking, "Is Beijing reached by taking an airplane or by taking a train?" This question makes no sense! There is only one Beijing, so if you get there, then you're there, regardless of whether you take trains or planes. That's how *taijiquan* is, too. If you can stay in the *taiji* state and apply the martial art while facing an opponent, then you have arrived at the destination. If you still cannot use *taijiquan* in combat, then you remain en route.

While en route, should you take the Chen boat, or the Yang boat? Either is fine. Before you've arrived, there is a difference between the Yang and Chen styles. After you arrive, there is just *taiji*. If anybody insists to you that there is a difference between Yang style and Chen style *taijiquan*, you can be certain that that person is speaking to you from atop the proverbial boat. He or she has yet to reach the other shore.

Paradoxically, although the conclusion implied by this analogy is that martial artistry is ultimately of little importance, the fact is

---

[28] *Taiji*, "太極," is a notion that will be explored throughout this book. The character *quan*, "拳," means "fist," and implies martial arts. Thus, *taijiquan* means "the martial art based upon understanding *taiji*."

that it is still very important. Martial training remains important because *taijiquan* is a necessary tool for those who hope to arrive at the *taiji* state. Nevertheless, *taijiquan* in and of itself is not the goal. One reason many people fail to excel in *taijiquan* is that they spend a lifetime working on the details of their martial arts forms, never realizing that the form is just a vessel that was built to take practitioners towards the goal of *taiji*. This is like spending one's whole life building a boat and comparing it with other shipwrights'. "Is my boat sturdy?" "Look how beautiful these streamlines I made are." "Your streamlines aren't as pretty as mine." "I used mahogany over there, and even a bit of rosewood over here." "That guy said he did a silver inlay, but some people even do gold inlays." A fool will make comparisons like these from dawn till dusk, never once thinking, "I just want to leave dry dock and sail to my destination." That said, while it is true that a boat need not be pretty, it still shouldn't leak. In the end, one must be particular about martial artistry, but not *too* particular. As long as one's vessel is seaworthy and sails straight and true, it is good enough.

Some people love to wonder, "Of the three generations of Yang family forms, whose was correct? If Yang Luchan got it right, then did Yang Banhou and Yang Chengfu train the martial art incorrectly? Or was it Yang Chengfu who was right, and his predecessors who were wrong?" These questions reflect the wrongheaded concerns of the uninitiated. In actuality, all three of those masters practiced the same martial art. Their individual physical constitutions, ways of practicing, ages, understandings of the philosophy and so forth were certainly distinct, and for these reasons differences were apparent in their martial arts forms. This is totally normal, and it does not mean that the essence changed.

The full name for *taijiquan* is "the thirteen forces of *taiji*."[29] *Taijiquan* forms are used to train in the ways of applying thirteen forces: *peng, lü, ji, an, cai, lie, zhou, kao, jin, tui, gu, pan,* and *ding*.[30] These

---

[29] This is "太極十三勢," with the final character, "勢," meaning "force."

[30] 掤, 捋, 擠, 按, 採, 挒, 肘, 靠, 進, 退, 顧, 盼, and 定.

names do not refer to a sequence of fancy moves, so they were not named the "thirteen movements of *taiji*." Even though my lineage's *taijiquan* form has eighty-eight movements, it is used only for training with these thirteen forces. One must understand this point to see beyond the superficial differences in sets of martial arts moves.

There are some martial arts enthusiasts who exclaim to me, "Did you know so-and-so can do all five styles of *taijiquan*?" This is a meaningless statement. One can take a boat today, switch to a car tomorrow, and later swap over to an airplane, but in the end it's still the same old person who arrives in Beijing. Misguided aspirants often end up practicing a hodgepodge of different martial arts, just as though they were wasting energy and resources to build a whole flotilla of boats, but never setting sail towards their destinations. This is a lamentable mistake.

I wish to draw readers' attention to these issues because, far from being rare, they constitute an extremely serious problem in the world of *taijiquan*. People are focused on comparing each *taijiquan* style's forms to see what the differences between them are, when in actuality there is nothing to compare. It is thus my frequent refrain that a major reason people do not train well is that people lack direction. That they lack direction is because they do not know what *taiji* really is.

A person who plans to master *taijiquan* by memorizing a few *taijiquan* forms is comparable to a person who says he or she would like to go to Beijing without even knowing what Beijing is! A person who thinks that having memorized a *taijiquan* form means he or she now understands *taiji* is as senseless as a person who takes a seat in a bus, car, or boat and announces that he or she has already arrived in Beijing. Beware of making this massive mistake.

# 3

# Martial Theory

*Explaining the key points in Wang Zongyue's*
Treatise on Taijiquan

*Wang Zongyue's original text*

*Taiji*. It is born of *wuji*. It is the mother of *yin* and *yang*. When it moves it divides, when tranquil it merges. Not exceeding, not insufficient, it follows that which curves and cleaves to that which straightens.

When others are hard and I am soft, this is called moving. When I follow behind others, this is called sticking. When movements are swift, I swiftly respond; when movements are slow, I slowly follow. Though changes are myriad, this principle is the one thing that threads through them all.

Go from increasing familiarity to gradually cognizing strength.[31] Go from understanding strength to arriving at wis-

---

[31] "Strength" here is from the character "勁" (often seen in its transliterated form as "*jin*" or "*jing*" in English writings on Chinese martial arts), not "力" (*li*). In discussion, Master Ren explained, "This is a reference to the principles by which strength is exerted. The 'strength' we seek to understand is not so much a thing as it is a principle. When one understands the principles of moving when *yin* and *yang* mutually nourish one another, then one has

dom,³² step by step. If you do not persistently exert yourself, you will be unable to suddenly comprehend that which connects to everything.

Emptily guide strength upwards, let *qi* sink to your *dantian*. Be not askew, be not awry; now hidden, now apparent. If your left is weighted, then your left is empty; if your right is weighted, then your right is traceless. Seen from below, you tower without end; seen from above, you are unendingly deep. The more others approach you, the further away you are; the more others retreat, the closer you follow. A single feather cannot be added, and a gnat finds nowhere to land. Others cannot fathom me—I alone know others. All heroes without match started here, and then they arrived!

The false doors leading away from such skill are numerous. Though they differ in form, none of these doors lead beyond the bullying of the weak by the strong and the capitulation of the slow to the quick. Those with strength pummel those without strength, slow hands succumb to fast hands—this all comes from ability we are born with, and is unrelated to that possessed by those whose strength is learned. Look at the phrase, "Use two hundred grams to uproot 500 kilograms"—it is obviously not strength that wins! Look at the physique of an octogenarian who can defend himself against a mob—how could he be quicker than they are?

As a balance scale stands or as a cart's wheel spins, if weight

---

begun to 'cognize strength.' One fully cognizes strength when one understands the laws of *yin* and *yang* as well as substantiality and insubstantiality."

³² "Wisdom" here comes from "神明." Master Ren explained his interpretation: "This wisdom transcends both body and mind, and its nature is to sense and affect that which is exterior to oneself, including other people. Daoists hold that this wisdom can exert itself beyond one's own body. After one trains to this level, this aspect of the teaching will become clearer and clearer. If one does not start by understanding *yin* and *yang* as well as substantiality and insubstantiality, then later there is no way to achieve this kind of wisdom. Gradually, as one reaches late stages in practice, one will start to experience strength that transcends the physical body."

falls on one side, then both sides move; but if weight falls on both sides, then both become stuck. Whenever you see one who has diligently trained for many years but cannot transform force, this is always this person's own fault—he or she has not comprehended the malady of double-weightedness.

If you wish to avoid this malady, you must know *yin* and *yang*. Sticking is moving, moving is sticking. *Yang* does not leave *yin*, *yin* does not leave *yang*. Only when *yin* and *yang* nurture one another do you understand strength.

After you comprehend strength, then the more you train the more you refine your skill. Silently contemplating and analyzing, eventually you are able to do as your heart wishes.

The foundation lies in giving up the self and following others. The common mistake is giving up the close and seeking the distant. That is called "a miniscule miscalculation that causes you to miss by a thousand miles." Students cannot but be finely discerning!

Such are my opinions.

## *An explanation of the* Treatise on Taijiquan

Wang Zongyue's *Treatise on Taijiquan* has been regarded as a classic by all practitioners of *taijiquan* for as long as it has existed.[33] Wang Zongyue bestowed it upon Jiang Fa, who then passed it on to Chen Changxing and Chen Qingping. It was later found in Jiang Fa's old rice store by Wu Yuxiang.

The teaching of *taijiquan* started with Zhang Sanfeng, who transmitted it to Wang Zongyue. Wang Zongyue transmitted *taijiquan* to Chen Changxing and Chen Qingping, who then passed it to the Yang and Wu families. The Yang and Wu lines constitute the earliest branches of *taijiquan*, which were then passed from the Wus to Hao Weizhen; Hao transmitted *taijiquan* to Sun Lutang, who created Sun

---

[33] Wang Zongyue's text is called 《太極拳論》 in Chinese.

style *taijiquan*. Wu Quanyou was a Manchu who studied martial arts with Yang Luchan and Yang Banhou. Later on his son, Wu Jianquan, developed Wu family *taijiquan* in Shanghai.[34]

In all, there are five main branches of *taijiquan*: Chen style, Yang style, Wu style, Wu style, and Sun style. The quintessential piece of writing for all of these styles is Wang Zongyue's *Treatise on Taijiquan*. Wu Yuxiang and Li Yishe also produced numerous treatises later on, but their theories on martial arts were simply permutations of Wang Zongyue's *Treatise*, and in many instances their essays were exegeses of Wang's original piece of writing.

Students of *taijiquan* need to clearly recognize that Wang Zongyue's *Treatise on Taijiquan* is the standard which determines whether you train correctly or not. If you conform to it, then you are training properly; if you are not in accord with it, then you're training incorrectly. There is nothing to be confused about—everything is measured against the *Treatise*. In the beginning, this was the very first criterion that my teacher gave me.

"*Taiji*. It is born of *wuji*, it is the mother of *yin* and *yang*."

This is the first sentence of the *Treatise on Taijiquan*. The first thing many people do when they read the *Treatise* is gloss over this sentence, because they think it is surely no more than meaningless boilerplate tacked onto the opening of the essay so that Wang would not appear unscholarly. Such assumptions are highly mistaken, and any martial artist who truly wishes to enter *taiji*'s gate needs to clearly understand what is being conveyed here.

*Taijiquan* theory comes from Daoist philosophy, which has two core principles: "the individual and all things merging as one" and

---

[34] This Wu style *taijiquan* is named after the surname "吴," while the branch identified above is named for the surname "武," both of which are written as "Wu" when Romanized.

"*yin-yang*-insubstantial-substantial."[35] The merging of an individual and all else in creation into oneness is called *"wuji."* *Wuji* is synonymous with *Qi*, and therefore it implies the total scope of your perception and experience. If you do not enter the treatise's teachings with this understanding, then you are ill-prepared for any general discussion of internal martial arts, and wholly unprepared for a discussion specific to *taijiquan*.

Daoists refer to "the universe and humanity becoming one"[36]—the state in which one's self, others, and all contained between heaven and earth become as though a single entity and merge with the Dao— as *wuji*. Some readers might feel compelled to retort, "But I am me, others are themselves, the sky is the sky, the ground is the ground, so how could they become a single entity?" In answer, what is meant is that if the heavens, the earth, others, and yourself are within the scope of your awareness all at once, then effectively these things are all one. Conversely, when you do not have them all within the realm of your perception at once, then the sky is the sky, the ground is the ground, others are themselves, and you are you alone.

The biggest error we can see people making when they push hands is this: the moment two people cross hands, they instantaneously recognize one another as opponents. This state of mind is far removed from *taiji*. In *taijiquan*, the very moment you and another person come face-to-face and cross hands, you must immediately merge with him or her. You become as though one, so that you may perceive each and every movement coming from the other person's body. You must allow every undulation of the other person's *shen* and *qi* to fall within the scope of your knowing. The *Treatise on Taijiquan* alludes to this when it says, "Others cannot fathom me—I alone know others. All heroes without match started here, and then they arrived!"

The starting point for training that will take you to the point of being unmatched under heaven lies in perceiving your opponents in

---

[35] The first principle is written "天人合一," while the second is written "陰陽虛實."

[36] This is an alternate translation of "天人合一."

their entirety. It really is possible to achieve "others cannot fathom me—I alone know others." If you have this skill, then in push hands, the instant you touch hands with another individual, that person will be unable to move his or her feet, let alone throw a punch. At the crucial moment when an opponent is on the cusp of lifting a foot or throwing a punch, you will already know what your opponent is trying to do, and deny him or her the opportunity. This is why Yang Luchan was able to place a bird on his palm and prevent it from taking flight. He most certainly did not have superglue on his palm. Rather, when the bird tried to push down with its legs in order to take flight, Master Yang dissipated its downwards-thrusting strength. The power of perception was the foundation of Yang Luchan's exquisite ability to transform and dissolve strength.

"Listening to strength" is one of the most important concepts in *taijiquan*.[37] This odd-sounding expression may elicit the question, "Why don't they call it 'feeling for strength?'" In actuality, the instruction is *not* to literally try and tune your ears into your sense of touch, as your sense of touch is clearly incapable of hearing. This somewhat abstruse *taijiquan* term is reminiscent of the instruction some Chan Buddhists give their students, to "listen to the clouds." Clouds are obviously something you can only see—why would a master tell a disciple to go and listen to them? The answer is that the real point of these instructions is to prevent practitioners from remaining stuck in old habits of perception. "Listen to the clouds" is an instruction to directly experience the actual state of the clouds instead of merely looking at their outward appearances. "Listening to strength" is the same.

In the practice of martial arts these are crucial concepts. If you are able to understand the concept of *wuji*, then you have already entered the proverbial door in your training. Even though their wording is abstract, I feel that these instructions have great practical value. Far too many practitioners do not start their training here.

---

[37] This literal translation of the term "聽勁" is common in the English-speaking *taijiquan* world.

"When it moves it divides, when tranquil it merges."

"When it moves it divides" refers to the division into *yin* and *yang*. "When tranquil it merges" refers to merger into *wuji*, the state of perceptive knowing, from which *yin* and *yang* emerge.

In the *taiji* symbol, we call the white area with a black spot *yang*, and we refer to the black area with a white spot as *yin*. Countless people have offered explanations of what *taiji* means, but in terms of describing what is needed to develop applicable martial skill, their explanations fail to satisfy me. My teacher, Dong Bin, once offered an explanation specifically from this standpoint. He said that the ancients used the famous *yin-yang* symbol in order to give a very panoramic, sweeping view of *taiji*. In the white area with a black dot, the white color represents a space in which there are no things, while the black dot is one's *shen* and one's thinking, which must remain vigilant.[38] In the black area with a white dot, the black portion represents a place where there are objects which have substance, while the white dot is one's *shen* and thoughts,[39] which should be empty and insubstantial.

Master Dong said that the *yin-yang* symbol implies that when pushing hands with another person, one must maintain emptiness in one's own body.[40] This will cause opponents to feel they have

---

[38] Of this vigilance, in discussion Ren said to me, "Your mind must be placed firmly upon what you are observing. *Qi* must be placed there. Pay full attention to what you are observing. Your mind must be right there."

[39] "*Shen* and thoughts" here comes from a compound of two Chinese characters, "神" and "意." This compound has no direct translation, so I have broken it into its components, transliterating one and translating the other. However, in conversation Master Ren emphasized that to the high level practitioner of *taijiquan* they are ultimately one, while stressing that an empty, receptive state must be maintained at all times in order for one to experience what is implied by these words.

[40] In discussion, Master Ren explained that with this type of emptiness, an opponent feels that one is both empty and impossible to grab ahold of—he or she finds no place on one's body upon which to exert strength. In order to

nothing to grasp ahold of. At the same time as one maintains internal emptiness, one's *shen* and *Qi* must also fill the space outside of one's body. Achieving this state is referred to as entering *taiji*. If a practitioner can succeed at doing so, a fight is already half won before any blows are thrown.

Doing authentic *taiji* means being able to make the space occupied by one's physical body empty, while filling the space beyond the physical body that falls within the scope of one's perception with one's *shen*. One must do this in such a way that *yang* does not separate from *yin* and *yin* does not separate from *yang*. The two must exist simultaneously. This state is named *taiji*.

Laozi's *Daodejing* describes this subjective state as "knowing the white and keeping watch on the black."[41] In this phrase, "keeping watch on the black" alludes to the requirement that one empty out the space occupied by one's body. One should not "know" this space, because if one does so, then this space will become as though a substantial entity—in terms of *taijiquan*, it will turn into a solid target for an opponent to attack. Thus, one must "know" the *yin-yang* symbol's white area, which represents the space beyond the physical borders of one's body. To Daoists, "knowing the white and keeping watch on the black" is the optimal condition for all objects and phenomena in the universe. For this reason, the criteria of *taiji* are also commonly applied to judge the merits of works of calligraphy and brush painting, and students of classical Chinese art are taught that "the place

---

demonstrate this principle, he had me push his arm. First he resisted, giving me a place to push against. Then he went soft, allowing me to push him around. Both resistance and softening reflected common mistakes. Finally he entered the "empty" state, and no matter how I pushed him, he constantly was able to get out of the way. The feeling was (to borrow Ren's words, which perfectly matched what I experienced) just like trying to push an object that is floating atop water. An object floating on water is constantly able to escape from one's grasp and move elsewhere whenever one pushes against it.

[41] The term "知其白, 守其黑" comes from the twenty-eighth chapter of the *Daodejing*. It is variously translated. Ren's commentary on this sentence is not intended as an "authoritative" interpretation of Laozi's original statement; it is specific to this context in *taijiquan*.

where ink settles must be empty and yet alive" while "the spaces the brush does not reach must brim with *qi*."

It is worth pausing here and reflecting upon a question: How many of us live up to these standards when we practice *taijiquan*?

> "Not exceeding, not insufficient, it follows that which
> curves and cleaves to that which straightens."

"Not exceeding and not insufficient" means that when one crosses hands with another person, one must never let one's hands exit the range of one's perception. When many people push hands, it is as though their bodies retreat into the background while only their hands remain in the foreground. When somebody does that, their hands have essentially already extended beyond their scope of perception.

"It follows that which curves and cleaves to that which straightens" means that, when both people in combat merge into a single entity and become a single field of *qi*, when one's opponent draws backwards, one's own *qi* continuously enters and fills the space the opponent has just vacated. This *taijiquan* method is extraordinarily useful during combat because few practitioners of other martial arts can do the same, much less counteract such action. Most martial artists either let their bodies deflate the moment they move their legs, or else let their legs deflate as soon as they try to move their torsos.[42]

---

[42] The characters Ren uses here are "瘪掉," which I have translated here as "deflate." In discussion he elaborated that this means to mistakenly relax in such a way that, should one's opponent use speed and strength to attack, he or she will be able to easily enter into one's own space. A person with *taijiquan* skill, therefore, avoids "deflation" and remains "full." When "full," as soon as the opponent uses speed or strength, the person skilled in *taijiquan* will automatically, spontaneously respond with equal speed and strength. Master Ren demonstrated this by having me try to make a sudden move against him; even though he was apparently standing in total relaxation, the moment my hand struck out towards his neck, his fist had already landed

When people with this habit move, their postures become imbalanced and they need to make small adjustments. If a person with a degree of skill in *taijiquan* spars with such a person, even if that person only needs to adjust for an instant, he or she will already have fallen behind the one who remains in the *taiji* state. It is extremely difficult for others to find the weak points of one who knows how to "follow that which curves and cleave to that which straightens." Herein lies the eminent practicability of *taijiquan*'s philosophical concept of merging into oneness!

> "When others are hard and I am soft, this is called moving. When I follow behind others, this is called sticking."

This sentence means that when one who is in the *taiji* state senses an opponent's strength, his or her body will respond to what has been perceived and correspondingly move to diffuse the opponent's strength.[43] This requires letting one's body move evenly in order to softly transform one's opponent's pressure. One must not block him or her by resisting or using raw strength. In the process of "moving," one's aim is also to repel one's opponent by having him or her discharge force and consequently fall into a trap wherein he or she can do nothing but passively submit to an attack. Facing an onslaught of force, the opponent will be incapable of throwing off the *taiji* practi-

---

painfully on my abdomen. Master Ren's explanation is that his state is like that of a loaded and cocked crossbow. Although the crossbow appears still, it ready to release a bolt at any time. All it took was my own movement to pull the trigger.

[43] When questioned by a reader of an early draft about my use of the word "moving" to translate the character "走" (which can literally mean "to walk" or "to run"), I asked Master Ren to explain the character to me yet one more time. He said that to "走" in the *Treatise* is akin to being in "a state of correspondence" ("相應的狀態") with one's opponent. Being in this "state of correspondence" naturally *produces* sticking, and leads one's opponent to fear letting down his or her guard.

tioner, and indeed will be too overwhelmed to even try. When this happens, it appears as though he or she were glued in place.[44]

Readers must be aware that moving and sticking, despite being discussed separately, are actually intrinsic components of a single concept. One does not first move and then stick, nor first stick and then move. To move is to store force. Once one's opponent falls into an empty space, naturally he or she will end up behind one's force and become stuck. Those who experience these things firsthand can be said to have "cognized strength."

> "When movements are swift, I swiftly respond;
> when movements are slow, I slowly follow."

What is described here is very easy to understand: when one's opponent is fast, one too is fast; when one's opponent is slow, one too is slow. Such accord is based upon skill in listening to strength.

If one's opponent uses 1 kg of strength, one should not use 1.1 kg, nor should one use 0.9 kg.[45] At the same time, one cannot try and guess how much force one's opponent is using. The only way to respond accurately is through direct perception. If one tries to guess, thinking "the other person is using about 0.15 kg of strength, so I'll use about 0.15 kg," accuracy is lost. One who practices *taijiquan* must sense an opponent while one's mind, *qi*, bones, and flesh are

---

[44] When I asked in person about this point, Master Ren demonstrated how it is not a question of some sort of trick that literally sticks the opponent in place. Rather, by using his *shen* and *Qi*, Ren made it so that I, in the role of his opponent, could not feel comfortable moving my body in any way. This discomfort stemmed from an uncanny and deeply unnerving sense of precarity.

[45] In discussion Master Ren explained to me that there is no mental work involved when this principle is enacted in push hands or combat. A skilled *taijiquan* practitioner intuitively knows the amount of strength to exert, and it naturally matches the amount of strength the opponent is exerting.

all merged in unity with him or her. Immediate and proportionate responses flow directly from sensing.

> "Though changes are myriad, this principle is the one thing that threads through them all."

By the time he arrives at this sentence, Wang Zongyue has already fully expressed the overarching theory of *taijiquan*. Now that he has told us how to practice, the subsequent content pertains only to methodology and analysis. The ideas introduced above in fewer than one hundred Chinese characters constitute the core principles of *taijiquan*. One could thus argue that *taijiquan* is not at all complicated, but scarce few people practice as Wang Zongyue prescribes. Unfortunately, instead of training in accordance with the *Treatise on Taijiquan*, most practitioners invent their own theories and practices.

Rumor has it that a few members of martial society wish to gather a handful of famous martial artists together and entreat each of them to write something poignant. The words of these luminaries will then be carved in stone and a "forest of steles" will be erected somewhere, with each of these teachers' remarks emblazoned on monoliths that people can come and appreciate in perpetuity. I am adamantly opposed to this proposal, because I am convinced that no contemporary master could word things better than the ancients did, nor possess an understanding of the martial arts that surpasses the ancients. It is far more likely that this forest of steles would just be a maze of confusion, waylaying legions of future cultivators. That would be a tragic turn of events.

> "Go from increasing familiarity to gradually cognizing strength. Go from understanding strength to arriving at wisdom, step by step."

These two sentences tell us that once we understand the above theories, we then need to practice. If we fail to practice, we will end up complaining, "I understood the ideas and I studied the methods, but when it came time to apply them I still ended up fighting the same way I always have." Training is required to remold what in China is called the "*qi* of habit."⁴⁶ Consider the following: if one goes from using a lamp that's turned on by pulling a chain to one with an on-off switch, for quite some time whenever one goes to turn on the new lamp one will fumble to find the chain before remembering it is no longer there. "Qi of habit" is simply a term for the normal tendency of a person to repeatedly do whatever feels the most natural.

It is possible that one trains well, but in a real fight, what comes out is the wild flailing and swinging of a back alley dustup. In other words, even though one may have learned better techniques, what is most familiar is still what one falls back upon under duress. Training must be allowed to ripen over time in order to establish new habitual *qi*. Once training in a new way of doing things is mature, then the incorrect methods that previously felt familiar will gradually come to feel strange. The same process occurs with any form of self-cultivation.

If the guiding principles of one's martial training are correct, then regardless of whether one is training alone or with a partner, one is always learning to intuit strength.⁴⁷ In partner training, two people use push hands to get a feel for how to keep *yang* from leaving *yin*

---

⁴⁶ The Chinese word is "習氣," a simple compound of "habit" and "*qi*."

⁴⁷ In Wang Zongyue's original text, what I translate as "cognizing strength" is "懂勁." Here in the commentary, instead of the verb "懂," Ren uses a different verb, "悟." This verb arguably has no direct corollary in English, although it can be used to describe epiphanies, gnosis, insight, intuition, internalization, comprehension, and even enlightenment. In conversation I asked Master Ren to elaborate and he said the following: "This has to do with experience. A student needs to start with faith in *taijiquan*'s theories in order to be willing to train, but what a beginner has is no more than blind faith. However, once a student learns to apply the methods, then blind faith will turn into genuine faith. The process of proving the truth of the teachings to ourselves is the process of 'intuiting.' In China we often say that 'intuiting'

and vice versa while under a degree of stress. One must be careful not to think that the goal of push hands is to shove the other person away or to put his or her arms and legs into some sort of lock. People who train push hands with such goals in mind end up cultivating half-baked shoving and grappling skills that are utterly useless in real fights.

Here I need to bring up another important question: Given that *taijiquan*'s philosophical principles are not terribly hard to grasp, why is it that in spite of understanding them people still don't practice well, and consequently fail to reach the levels of practitioners of days gone by?

One of the primary reasons is laziness! In the past, our predecessors, including my teacher, would always say: "Your martial arts form can only be considered mature if you've trained it 10,000 times!" Thus, if one's dream is to complete one's training in a year and a half, one would have to practice a *taijiquan* form more than twenty times a day. In reality, how many times do we really train our forms each day? When training intensely, three sessions in a single day already counts as pretty good. When not intensely focused, one realistically might do the form twice a day. It is extremely hard to reach the ancients' level by training like this. This is an area that demands martial artists to improve our self-knowledge and perform introspection.

Early on I discussed the problems of martial arts training with my teacher. He said that when we first start, we learn an entire form, and at minimum we need to train with it a thousand times in order to move beyond the stage of always wondering, "Should my hands be higher or lower? Should my legs be closer together or farther apart? When I move my hands in this direction should they make one circle or two?" After training the form a thousand times or so, these thoughts will lose their relevance because one's musculature will have already developed deep-rooted habits. Only at this stage,

---

must be done via the body. When rooted in bodily experience, intuition is not simply a matter of mental activity. In fact, it transcends mental activity."

where the mind begins to quiet down, does it become practical to go on to intuit strength, which means physically intuiting the concepts of *wuji* and *taiji* that we discussed earlier.

The process of intuiting or cognizing strength begins naturally once one has trained a *taijiquan* form approximately one thousand times. How this process unfolds is a key factor in determining whether or not one will enter the gate leading to the path of *taijiquan*. A degree of destined affinity is required for one to cognize strength.

Some people need only hear an excellent teacher offer a few instructions and make a demonstration in order to understand. I have encountered such people, and among my students such talents exist. However, people like this tend to be fairly lazy—thinking that *taiji* is easy to master with just a little study, they don't apply themselves to strenuous training, and in the end they're not even skilled enough to acquit themselves in a little shoving match between family members.

Some people are quite slow, and even after three or five years of practice it is an open question as to whether or not they will ever really understand *taijiquan*. I also have this sort of student. After practicing for several years and still not cognizing strength, one of them said to me, "Training with you is like playing cards. If I don't come to class, then I'm afraid that maybe that will be the day I was going to be dealt a really good hand. But even if I do come, I often go home dead broke. Frankly, I just don't understand what you're trying to teach us." However, recently he has begun to feel he like finally has a few good cards in his hand, so he is developing confidence and the *taijiquan* teachings are beginning to play out in his own body. In short, while training is of paramount importance, because the ability to cognize strength is determined in part by intuition, it cannot be sweated into existence.

There is another pass that needs to be traversed after one is able to intuit strength, that of ripening. Having intuitive epiphanies will allow one to clearly understand new principles and methods of applying strength, but how does one bring this understanding to maturity? At this stage, one must, at minimum, train one's *taijiquan* form another 4,000 times, after which point it will be "ripe." My teacher Dong Bin's requirement was to train the form an additional 10,000 times *after* learning to intuit strength. I personally no longer have such a stringent requirement, as I realize that if I required people to train the form more than 10,000 times, all of my students would scatter to the wind. If I only require students to train the form 5,000 times, there might be a few people who will keep chipping away.

While I do require students to practice the form 5,000 times, I do not say to them that they must finish within a year and a half or two years. In my opinion, that is too difficult for people with modern lifestyles to accomplish. However, recently I suggested to a friend that if the opportunity arises we should take on some young students living in a remote area and set up a foundation to cover their monthly expenses, so that they can train rigorously while free of worries about making money. If they trained like this for five to eight years, their accomplishments would be incredible!

> "If you do not persistently exert yourself, you will be unable to suddenly comprehend that which connects to everything."

When Wang Zongyue speaks of "that which connects to everything," he means that once one's practice has matured, one will thoroughly understand the principles that prevent *yin* and *yang* from separating when one is in the fray of a fight. When one's body first begins to understand what this concept means, one has just begun "cognizing strength." If one persists in training, one's skills will progressively ripen, and one will eventually come to feel one's hands working in marvelous ways when pushing hands. One's body will also become increasingly capable of doing precisely what the mind commands. However, without stringent training, it will remain very difficult to have the sort of sudden epiphany that ties everything together.

This brings us to the end of our discussion of the principal theories presented by Wang Zongyue in his *Treatise on Taijiquan*. Terms below like "emptily guide strength upwards" and "let *qi* sink to your *dantian*" refer only to specific training methods.

> "Emptily guide strength upwards,[48] let *qi* sink to your *dantian*.
> Be not askew, be not awry; now hidden, now apparent.
> If your left is weighted, then your left is empty;
> if your right is weighted, then your right is traceless"

What we will discuss going forward are some of the fundamental requirements for martial arts training. The first sentence reads, "emptily guide strength upwards, let *qi* sink to your *dantian*." There are major errors in many people's interpretations of this sentence. The most common and most grievous error lies in attempts to understand emptily guiding strength upwards and letting *qi* sink to the *dantian* by breaking the two ideas apart. That is a massive mistake, as these two instructions are in fact two sides of the same coin.

What "emptily guiding strength upwards" refers to is gently raising the body, as though from head to toe there exists a central line that raises the whole body. When Qi is relaxed, ancestral *qi* will naturally sink down into the *dantian*.[49] Nowadays, the majority of *taijiquan* practitioners adopt a stance that is nothing like this when they push hands or train forms. When pushing hands, the first thing they do is either deeply bend at the knees, or else force their abdomens downwards. Because they wildly misinterpret the notion of "sinking *qi* into

---

[48] In conversation Master Ren said that this should be understood as straightening and lifting the position of one's head in an empty (light and non-forceful) manner.

[49] Ancestral *qi*, a term students of Chinese medicine will recognize, is written as "宗氣." Master Ren explained to me that this is *qi* in the body which should naturally flow downwards. It is produced by the body in the thoracic (膻中) area and flows downwards to the "sea of *qi*" or "氣海" region, which is just beneath the belly button and related to (but not synonymous with) the lower *dantian*. Ren called this the "foremost *qi*" of the body.

the *dantian*," they believe that doing these things will firmly stabilize their center of gravity. But really, if one pauses to think about it, that is not letting *qi* sink into the *dantian*—that's jamming *qi* down into the *dantian*!

Misinterpreting a single word can ruin everything. When one's stance is like what I just described, one is categorically incapable of "emptily guiding strength upwards."⁵⁰ From the standpoint of *taijiquan* this is catastrophic, because simultaneously emptily guiding strength upwards while letting *qi* sink to the *dantian* is precisely what is required in this martial art. The *dantian* only fills as *qi* naturally settles downwards. A person's being able to stand stock still with three people trying to push him or her over is not evidence that *qi* has

---

⁵⁰ A reader expressed confusion with my way of using "emptily guiding strength upwards" to translate "虛領頂勁" (which is sometimes written in Chinese as "虛靈頂勁", although Master Ren asked me *not* to use the latter configuration and had me remove it from the Chinese version of the *Treatise* I based my translation on). Indeed, what I can offer to the reader is only an imperfect translation of four characters that describe the nearly-ineffable in such vague terms that endless ink has already been spilled in native Chinese speakers' attempts to explain them to other native speakers! Worried that there might be a major problem with my translation, I asked Master Ren to clarify the term for me one more time. Echoing what is said many times in this book, he explained that this term does not refer to the head guiding *qi*, a way of pushing, or any other specific action. Rather, it refers to a strength that develops from the bottom of the body up through to the top, finally giving a practitioner a unified, central axis. This central axis develops from the waist, gradually comes to include the thorax, and finally encompasses even the crown of the head. It develops in those who consistently embrace a state where the body is blended with the space around it when they practice *taijiquan*. Once this axis and its *qi* reach to the top of the head (after a long period of training likely spanning many years), a practitioner's body moves in an empty, alive, and united manner that bestows uncanny strength. Conversely, if one has not "emptily lifted *qi*" all the way to the top of the head (again, Master Ren emphasized that this is not a discrete action but a *result* of proper practice), then the strength one can command when attempting to use *taijiquan* in combat or push hands will be far less than what it could be. Another way to translate "虛領頂勁" is "emptily guide the strength that envelops your entire body all the way to the top of your head."

sunk into the *dantian*. Rather, it simply shows that this person knows how to mash *qi* down into the *dantian*.

The next sentence reads, "be not askew, be not awry." When a fighter is neither askew nor awry, his or her body can freely move, transform an opponent's strength, or strike. However, this instruction is useless if it is not predicated by the previous instruction to simultaneously "emptily guide strength upwards" and "sink *qi* to the *dantian*," because if this requirement has not been fulfilled, then the *taijiquan* fighter will have no strength to expel.

Many people who train martial arts use the horse stance as their foundation, but how many of them train it correctly? When most people train the horse stance, they jam themselves in one place and squat very low. What, precisely, is equestrian about this stance? This has nothing to do with any horse! The horse stance has its name because it should evoke the state of a horseman in ancient times riding a steed into battle. Consider: could one really squat low like so many martial artists do while actually riding on horseback? As soon as the horse broke into a gallop, one would plonk up and down so miserably that one's intestines would be squeezed right out! That's why when people ride horses they hold fast with their groins. A rider's waist should raise his or her legs, which should squeeze against the horse's sides. This way, if the rider were to wield a massive saber or a lance, he or she would be able to connect the weapon in his or hands with the force of the horse's gallop and use the two in tandem to smite the adversary with a staggering blow. Now consider: if one were to use that mistaken squatting posture to ride horseback while trying to attack enemies with a saber or a lance, one would be in a sorry state long before reaching the enemy line. Thus, in *taijiquan* we start by training the waist, in order to learn to lift our legs from our waists.

These days one hears certain voices stating that people should avoid *taijiquan* because a lot of practitioners ruin their knees. As soon as an elderly person says he or she is practicing *taijiquan*, some doctor will sternly warn, "Stop practicing, otherwise you'll destroy your knees." Are these doctors speaking without having any idea what they're talking about? Not at all—indeed lots of people do harm their knees through practice. However, this does not mean that there is something inherently wrong with *taijiquan*. The crux of the matter is that people who harm themselves with *taijiquan* are not really practicing *taijiquan*.

The first physical requirement in *taijiquan* is to train the waist. *Taijiquan* does *not* ask students to press their centers of gravity down into their knees and feet. If it did, then as soon as people reached a certain age this sort of exercise would indeed become deleterious. Authentic Chinese martial arts do not work this way. Rather, they require that one uses one's waist to raise the entire body, so that one moves as though one's legs were dangling from the waist. Skilled practitioners do not use their legs to prop up their waists from below.

Another thing many *taijiquan* practitioners say nowadays is that their waists govern their bodies. But careful observation of their movements reveals that this is not the case! Wherever their feet go their waists follow, so how could their waists be in charge? Leading from the waist means that when the waist dictates where to move, the whole body acts in concert with it. When this is being done, the legs are no more than the waist's assistants.

The next line in the *Treatise* also cannot be embodied by a practitioner using flawed training methods. The next line states, "If your left is weighted, then your left is empty; if your right is weighted, then your right is traceless."[51] This is impossible to do unless one can emptily guide strength upwards and let *qi* sink to the *dantian*. Only when that instruction is mastered will a practitioner "stand like a balance scale," instead of instinctually bracing his or her body when faced with an opponent's strength.[52] Resisting is always incorrect, because

---

[51] Master Ren's book contains a parenthetical which states "'traceless' here also means empty." I wish to add that in discussion Ren made it very clear to me that "double weightedness" does *not* refer to the two sides of one's own body, and rather refers to one's own weight and that of one's opponent. In this context, the word "weight" actually refers to the exertion of strength.

[52] I discussed this point in detail with Master Ren. He said that the *Treatise*'s teaching on being like a balance scale comes from the fact that when a weight

a person who is stiffly braced cannot maintain balance while moving like a balance scale.

Thus, one must raise one's body, let *qi* settle into the *dantian*, and then treat Qi as a wheel and the waist as its axle. When one does this, one's body becomes just like a wheel. It is crucial to note that in question here is not the body's *qi*, but the primordial *qi* written as "Qi." One should also let one's *shen* be like the wheel on a cart, and one's waist be as though its axle. Readers must be cautious not to interpret these points as though they pertained to the *qi* inside of the human body. If one's thinking is limited in this way, then there is no way for "Qi to become a wheel." Conversely, if one succeeds at having *qi* sink into the *dantian* and emptily raising one's strength, then one's "wheel" will be incredibly responsive.

Those who say that many of the "ten requirements" for *taijiquan* were added onto the art by later practitioners are not mistaken.[53] All of them evolved from the phrases "emptily guiding strength upwards" and "*qi* sinking to the *dantian*," and therefore in no way supersede those basal instructions. Students should be cautious not to let instructions like these get in the way of the core teachings. For example, when applying the common *taijiquan* instruction to "hang the shoulders and sink the elbows," one must not actually let one's body hang downwards in any way.[54] My teacher often used to say

---

is placed on one arm of a balance scale, its other arm will automatically go up. A person who is stiffly braced because he or she is offering an opponent resistance is like a rusty balance scale. Even if one places a very heavy weight on a balance scale whose pivot has rusted shut, its arms will not move up or down (and a heavy enough weight will bring the whole structure crashing down!).

[53] According to Ren, these "requirements" (called "太極拳十要" in Chinese) can be found in writings by Yang Chengfu and Chen Weiming. He asked me to not detail them in this book, as he believes that more often than not these sorts of lists distract people from the essential teachings.

[54] In discussion Master Ren clarified that a person who understands *taijiquan* never "lifts up the shoulders," and this remains true even when his or her arms or shoulders actually *are* physically raised. The key to this apparent paradox is that because a *taijiquan* adept's arms, shoulders, body, and waist

that when one is training martial arts it should be as though one has two steamed bread rolls held beneath one's armpits. When we look at ancient paintings of people—especially those from the Tang dynasty and earlier—we see that the human figures seem to be floating upwards, if not outright taking flight. When you see buddhas depicted like that you feel reverence. Why? Because they seem to be uplifted by *Qi*.

Long ago, all educated people and government officials used to have to engage in the study and practice of *Qi*, which meant that almost everybody had a certain amount of skill and understood that people feel most comfortable when in a state of union with all things. However, as soon as the Song dynasty ended, figures depicted in art began to look flat.

---

are never separate, even though he or she may *appear* to be lifting his or her shoulders, this movement is still coming directly from the waist.

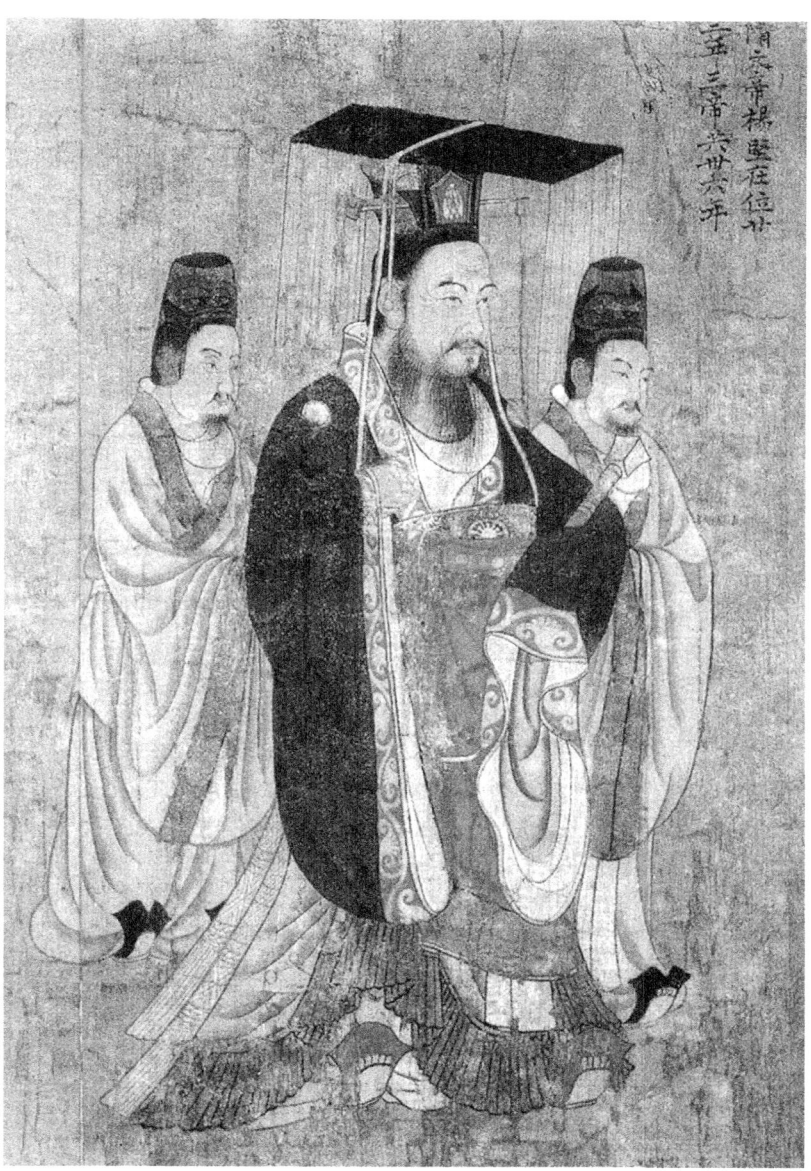

Portrait of King Wen of the Sui dynasty, attributed to Yan Lipen, 7th century

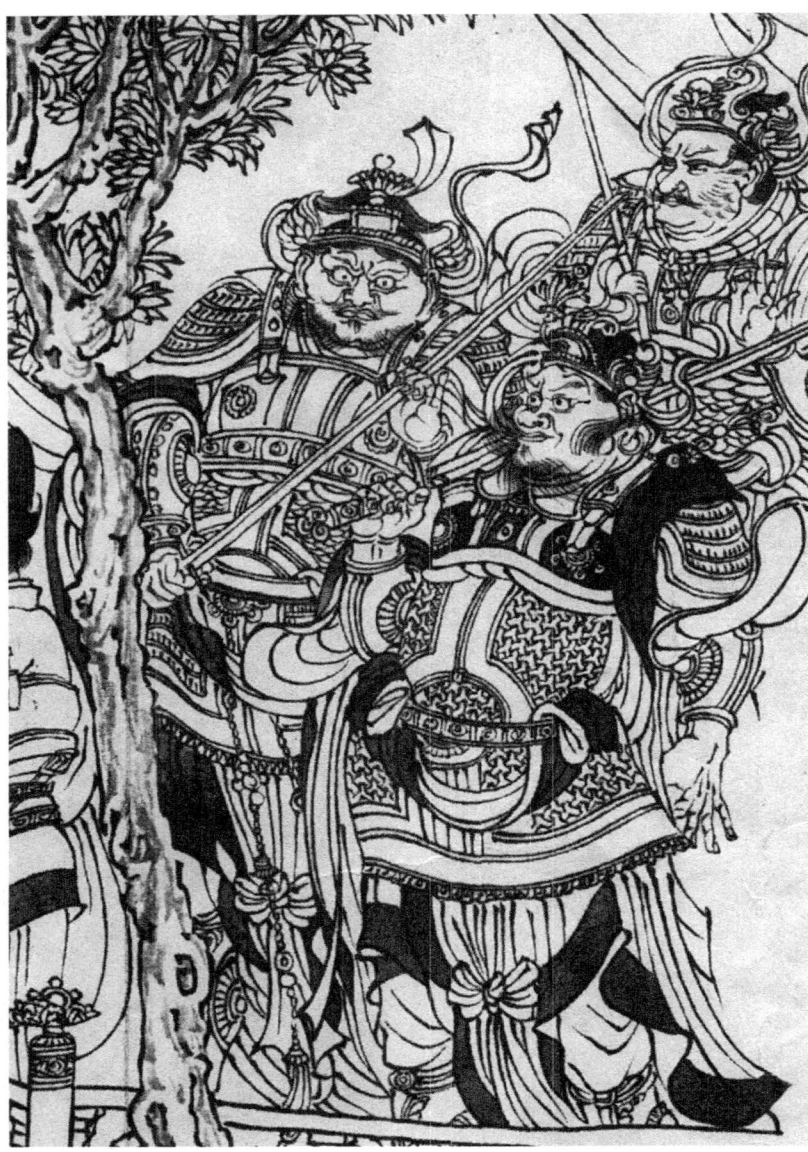

A detail from a Tang dynasty scroll entitled "The Eighty-seven Celestials." Its exact date and creatorship are unsettled.

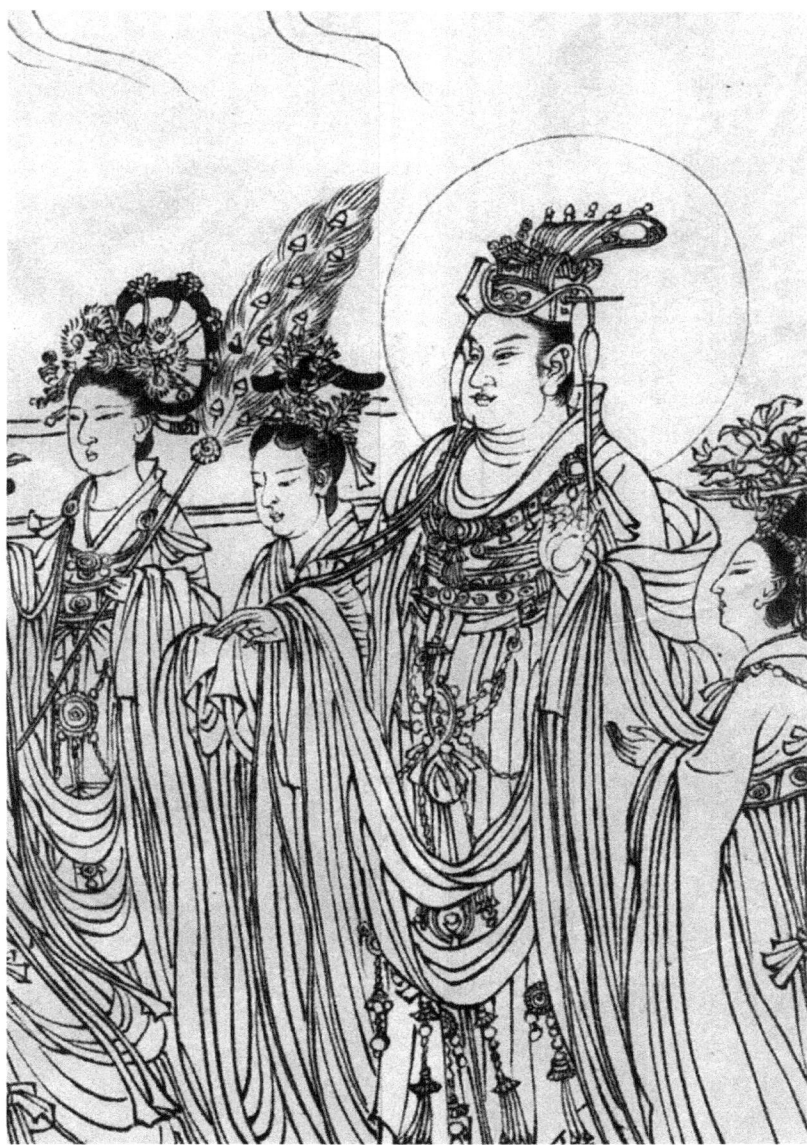

This detail also comes from "The Eighty-seven Celestials." Master Ren selected this image and the portrait of King Wen in order to illustrate the way in which ancient aesthetics were informed by *Qi* cultivation.

Take a look at ancient copper vessels—especially those from the Shang and Zhou dynasties, which are truly excellent—and how the shapes of these vessels all, metaphorically speaking, "raised their waists." The underlying reasons for China's great prosperity through the Tang dynasty are implied in its art. The feeling imbued in ancient copper vessels gives one the sense that there was no foreign army that could have conquered China back then. On the other hand, when one looks at the dainty items that became popular in the Song and Ming dynasties, one senses that they lack Qi and that they reflect a culture that is susceptible to bullying. More than being a simple matter of style, these changes reflect a society and culture's gradual loss of the knowledge of Qi.

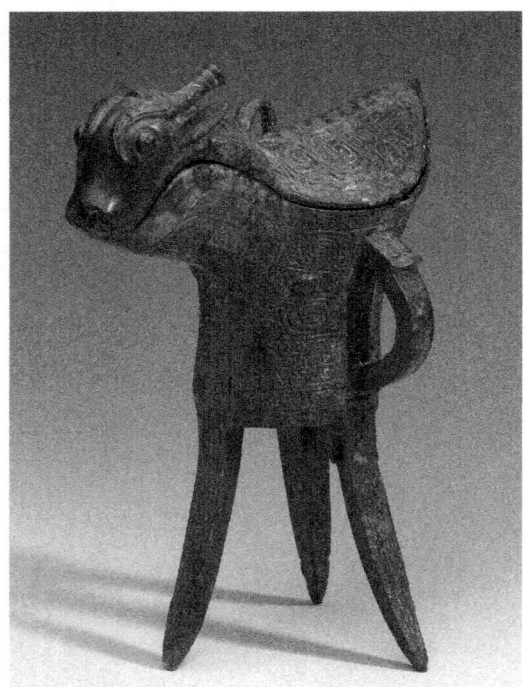

A bronze vessel for holding alcohol dating to the late Shang dynasty (c. 1600 BC – c. 1046 BC). Like the paintings above, this vessel's design suggests the movements of Qi that Master Ren describes in this book. From the collection of the National Palace Museum in Taiwan.

The waist is something I think people should pay special attention to. When our waists are elevated, the burden on our legs becomes very light, and people will remark how nimble we seem to be on our feet. There has to be strength in the waist in order for the legs to become agile. Practitioners of Chinese wrestling have numerous methods of training lumbar strength, so naturally they are very nimble on their feet.[55] Moreover, there is no way to defeat a Chinese wrestler by sinking low into an immobile horse stance. Any martial artist with this habit would be swiftly humiliated by most grapplers. A lightweight female judo practitioner can easily throw a much larger man who does not know how to use his body.

Once again, authentic *taijiquan* definitely does not harm the knees. Its leg and waist movements should actually improve the health and functioning of one's knees, legs and feet. Some time ago a professor in the United States named Tingsen Xu[56] published a compelling article on how to use *taijiquan* training to prevent trips and falls in the elderly. His research indicated that, at the very least, if one regularly trains waist and leg strength while maintaining balance, one will reinforce the joints as well as greatly reduce the chances of suffering from a fall.

> "Seen from below, you tower without end; seen from above, you are unendingly deep. The more others approach you, the further away you are; the more others retreat, the closer you follow."

Many people's interpretations of this passage are quite contrived. What it means is that if one is in the *taiji* state, "emptily guiding strength upwards" and "letting *qi* sink into the *dantian*," then one will be able to make an opponent who lies within the range of one's

---

[55] What I translate as "Chinese wrestling" is called "摔跤" in Mandarin and sometimes known by its *pinyin* name, "*shuaijiao*."
[56] Dr. Tingsen Xu, PhD, taught *taijiquan* to Jimmy Carter.

perception feel the following: "Seen from below, you tower without end; seen from above, you are unendingly deep. The more others approach you, the further away you are; the more others retreat, the closer you follow."

When I am pushing hands with another person, his or her range of motion lies within the scope of my perception, so from my perspective there is no question of high or low to speak of. When I am freely sparring with other people, they are also in the scope of my perception, so they only ever feel that the parts of my body they wish to strike are out of reach, and yet that I can make contact with their bodies in an instant. My force is always enveloping them, and yet they cannot grasp it. If they retreat, they cannot shake me. If they try to go high, there's no getting above me. If they try to go low, there's no getting beneath me.

Wang Zongyue's above passage discusses the range of one's force. These sentences extend from the philosophical concept of *taiji*, and therefore must be interpreted within this context in order to be understood correctly.

> "A single feather cannot be added,
> and a gnat finds nowhere to land."

"A single feather cannot be added, and a gnat finds nowhere to land" is a teaching on the authentic method of training. Success in *taijiquan* is not a measure of one's physical strength relative to others'. Success is a matter of cultivating the scope of one's perception. While practicing, one should make it so that a feather could not be placed upon one's body without one's knowing, and such that if a fly were to try to land on one's arm, one would perceive it, respond, and give the fly nothing solid to attach to.

While *taijiquan* really does have to be trained like this, let us first set aside the question of gnats. If one is being shoved by an actual *person*, it is imperative that one be capable of remaining dynamic!

My grand-teacher, Dong Shizuo, once lamented, "The *Treatise on Taijiquan* clearly explains 'a single feather cannot be added, and a gnat finds nowhere to land,' and yet plenty of *taijiquan* practitioners could do no more than stand stock still even if knives and hatchets were raining down on them, thinking, 'at least my center is very solid, I'm still not moving!'" *Taijiquan* students who train for this sort of misguided heroism are everywhere.

> "Others cannot fathom me—I alone know others. All heroes without match started here, and then they arrived!"

This sentence is a summary, reiterating that if one accomplishes "emptily guiding strength upwards" and "*qi* sinking to the *dantian*"— and, moreover, the scope of one's *taiji* and the scope of one's force are sufficiently expansive—then one will be able to make opponents feel that "seen from below, you tower without end; seen from above, you are unendingly deep. The more others approach you, the further away you are; the more others retreat, the closer you follow." Upon this foundation, if one knows how to keenly listen to force, then "a feather cannot be added and a gnat has nowhere to land."

The central goal of training is to have all of one's opponents' movements fall within the scope of one's knowledge and awareness, whilst one's opponents remain incapable of knowing what one is doing. If one's opponents lack highly refined powers of perception and cannot use *taijiquan*'s methods, then they will be unable to make any encroachments. This is what is implied by, "All heroes without match started here, and then they arrived." Naturally, this sentence does not imply that if one trains this way today, then tomorrow one will be a peerless warrior. Rather, it identifies the proper starting point.

My teacher, Dong Bin, often used to comment that when many people push hands, the person being pushed will bend backwards without letting his or her feet budge, as though to show how supple his or her waist is. There are others who stand there and brace themselves, so that even five people would struggle to push them over. Of such people he would chuckle and then say, "You should go up and try to slap them across the face, to see if they can parry or not. If they can't, then is that what you'd call a martial art? If they can stop people from pushing them over, well and good, but if enemies come at them with knives, will they just remain motionless? If all a practitioner can do is stand firm, then how is what they practice a martial art? All of that is for show; it's got nothing to do with authentic martial arts and *taiji* philosophy."

> "The false doors leading away from such skill are numerous. Though they differ in form, none of these doors lead beyond the bullying of the weak by the strong and the capitulation of the slow to the quick. Those with strength pummel those without strength, slow hands succumb to fast hands—this all comes from ability we are born with, and is unrelated to that possessed by those whose strength is learned."

"False doors" refers to mistaken training methods. People who train incorrectly are plentiful, and while each of them may harbor different misconceptions of the essence of martial arts, Wang Zongyue summarizes them all when he says, "None of these doors lead beyond the bullying of the weak by the strong and the capitulation of the slow to the quick. Those with strength pummel those without strength, slow hands succumb to fast hands." Admittedly, it is extremely difficult *not* to make these mistakes. When I'm pushing hands with my students I often say to them, "Hit me! But I want you to hit me in a way that does not come from relying upon greater strength to strike somebody of lesser strength, nor from relying on speed to try and hit somebody who is slower than you are." This is actually very hard to do! Many of my students are very strong, so when they are not careful what comes out is just strength, not actual *taijiquan* ability.

When Wang Zongyue says, "this all comes from ability we are born with, and is unrelated to that possessed by those whose strength is learned," he is referring to relying on attributes of our physical endowments—such as raw strength and speed—instead of mindfully acting in accord with the principles of *taiji*. Learning to effectively use brute strength and move quickly will help one win fights, but it ultimately has nothing to do with *taijiquan*'s requisite methods of using strength.

> "Look at the phrase, 'Use two hundred grams to uproot 500 kilograms'—it is obviously not strength that wins! Look at the physique of an octogenarian who can defend himself against a mob—how could he be quicker than they are?"

The genuine skill of using two hundred grams to uproot five hundred kilograms is clearly not something that is accomplished by relying on strength, because if it were, a *taijiquan* practitioner could not pull this off without sacrificing the nimble agility characteristic of this art. A lot of people say that using two hundred grams to uproot five hundred kilograms is no more than a clever trick, but they are mistaken. It is actually a way of transforming strength.

A subtle point that some of my elders recently brought to my attention is that the so-called "uprooting of five hundred kilos with two hundred grams" does *not* mean that when a person applies strength to one's body, one then uses a clever trick to redirect that strength somewhere else. Rather, it means that because one's body and the space around it are all moving with even force, one is therefore able to add one's opponent's force to the force of one's own body (which is not simply strength), and then to dissolve it or transform it within one's own body, or even to have it be evenly received by the space around oneself. This way, the strength one uses at the point of physical contact becomes extremely small, causing one's opponent to feel a sort of "empty" sensation. This empty sensation is called "transforming." If I was to say that my method of using strength was to divert incoming force, then that would be called "transferring," not "transforming."[57] What authentic *taijiquan* always teaches is the latter, not the former.

*Taijiquan* does not teach us to yield, it only teaches us to transform. My grand-teacher, Yue Huanzhi, said that there is no concept of "getting out of the way" in *taijiquan*.[58] My teacher, Dong Bin, once wrote me a letter, the gist of which was that when fighting one should feel as though one were letting one's opponent perform a full body search without offering any physical or mental resistance. In a fight it is often sufficient to simply transform all of an opponent's force until it is gone, because once one has transformed it into oblivion, no more threat to one's person remains. In fact, an opponent's force can flow right through one's own body. As students of *taijiquan*, we should be seeking to enter precisely this realm of skill and experience.

The next line asks, "Look at the physique of an octogenarian who can defend himself against a mob—how could he be quicker than they are?" Here arises an important question: is *taijiquan* fast or not? The answer is yes, but the caveat to that answer is that, in the context of *taijiquan*, speed refers to being able to move the body just as the mind wills. When learning *taijiquan*, in the beginning one "uses the mind to move *qi*," but ultimately, once there is real achievement, "the body is able to follow the mind." Speed in *taijiquan* comes from the body's unhindered ability to follow the mind—as soon as the mind moves somewhere, the body arrives with it.

---

[57] This distinction relates to the demonstration that Ren gave me for the note above, when he showed how "an opponent feels that you are both empty and impossible to grab ahold of—he or she finds no place on your body upon which to exert strength." I clarified with him that the "transforming" discussed here, from the Chinese character "化," happens spontaneously and effortlessly. Conversely, what I translate here as "transferring" (from "變") requires effort and applied technique.

[58] In person, Master Ren said to me that in China it is a common misconception that *taijiquan* teaches people to become very skilled at evasion.

In a fight, a *taijiquan* master does not try to anticipate or prepare for the opponent's next move by preemptively extending a hand or anything like that. Such movements are far too slow. Real alacrity as I am describing here comes as a natural product of regular practice. After the process of "ripening" we discussed earlier has unfolded and one's body now responds the moment the mind moves, this stage of training is accomplished. One's body must move with the mind if one wishes to progress from ripening to "wisdom."

So, when Wang Zongyue asks, "Look at the physique of an octogenarian who can defend himself against a mob—how could he be quicker than they are," although he implies that *taijiquan* mastery is not a question of physical speed, he does not mean that *taijiquan* is not fast. *Taijiquan* practitioners have a beloved refrain, "When my opponent is motionless, I don't move; when my opponent makes the slightest movement, I'm already in motion."[59] People who say this are talking about speed, but only about the very specific type of speed that lets the hands move the instant the mind does. The subtext of this statement is an instruction to not think, because thinking happens very slowly.

Thus, one with real skill throws a fist without *knowing* what is happening. In one important essay on *taijiquan* it is said, "I am not aware of how my hands are dancing, I do not know how my feet move."[60] At that level of skill, when the mind moves these things just emerge. There is no room for a fighter to stand there thinking about how to do things. When in combat, if one is concerned about how an opponent will attack and how one should respond, there is only a slim chance of success.

When using *taijiquan* in combat, winning or losing is not decided by the swiftness or lack thereof in one's fists and feet. Winning comes from the *taiji* state. *Taijiquan* training will not prepare a student for a

---

[59] From "彼不動我不動，彼微動我先動."

[60] From "不知手之所舞，足之所蹈." This phrase traces back to the "Record on the Subject of Music" or 〈樂記〉, a piece of writing on music and poetics included in the *Book of Rites* or 《禮記》.

simple contest of hand and foot speed; if I was to compete with other martial artists in this, I would undoubtedly be slower than those who do speed training every day. However, what I can do is see what kind of state my opponent occupies, and it is his or her state that I am capable of controlling. To do so, I perceive an opponent's force and gauge where his or her flaws lie. This skill is the marrow of the Chinese martial arts.

> "As a balance scale stands or as a cart's wheel spins, if weight falls on one side, then both sides move, but if weight falls on both sides, then both become stuck."

The phrase "as a balance scale stands or as a cart's wheel spins" illustrates how the *qi* of the *Treatise on Taijiquan* is definitely not the *qi* our bodies derive from foodstuffs, and rather is the *Qi* that comes from *wuwei*.⁶¹ If the *qi* Wang Zongyue is concerned with was the *qi* our bodies produce from food, he would not present the image of "spinning like a cart's wheel."

A lot of people have gone to great lengths trying to explain "if weight falls on one side, then both sides move, but if weight falls on both sides, then both become stuck," but what it implies is actually incredibly simple. This idea is connected to the sentences before it. "To stand like a balance scale" is synonymous with the prior instruction to stand with one's *qi* sinking to one's *dantian* while emptily guiding strength upwards; the prior instruction to have one's body

---

⁶¹ The Chinese character for "later heaven *qi*" is "氣," which contains the radical for rice (米) and can be interpreted as implying the energy that our bodies obtain from foods. Conversely, "prior heaven *Qi*" (炁) has no physical corollary and does not become accessible to us through any gross process—cooking, digestion, or otherwise—and thus Ren associates it with *wuwei*, a term from the *Daodejing* that can be translated as "non-doing." In conversation Ren emphasized to me that there must be an absence of thought for one to enter *wuwei* and access *Qi*.

be so alive that neither a feather nor a fly could settle on it is synonymous with "rotating like a cart's wheel."

"If weight falls on one side, then both sides move, but if weight falls on both sides, then both become stuck" means that when encountered with an opponent's force one will move just like the arm of a well-oiled balance scale which tips the moment a weight is placed upon it. Being able to do this means being able to follow an opponent. Conversely, if one falls into double-weightedness, then as soon as one encounters another's strength one fights against it, like a balance scale whose pivot is rusty. Such a balance scale possesses neither sensitivity nor accuracy.

Lots of people render the *Treatise on Taijiquan* impenetrable by treating its statements as though they were highly esoteric, but what Wang Zongyue says here is very clear and uncomplicated. No matter what some people might think, this is really a very simple text. To recapitulate what has been said thus far, the core instruction is to emptily guide strength upwards and let *qi* sink into the *dantian*. The additional instruction to remain as lively as a wheel means that as soon as one is touched by an opponent, one "listens." This is also called "letting go of self and following others." The instant one listens, one moves. If one fails to understand this, then one will resist when an opponent applies strength, which is called being "double-weighted." When one is double-weighted, it is impossible to make changes. In Wang Zongyue's analogy, being double-weighted means being like a broken balance scale.

> "Whenever you see one who has diligently trained for many years but cannot transform force, this is always this person's own fault—he or she has not comprehended the malady of double-weightedness. If you wish to avoid this malady, you must know *yin* and *yang*. Sticking is moving, moving is sticking. *Yang* does not leave *yin*, *yin* does not leave *yang*. Only when *yin* and *yang* nurture one another do you understand force."

Wang Zongyue observed that many people remain incapable of transforming opponents' strength in combat despite having trained for years, which leaves them at their opponents' whims. This happens because failing to internalize the concept of double-weightedness makes it impossible for people to eliminate the flaws in their fighting techniques. "If you wish to avoid this malady, you must know *yin* and *yang*" means that if one hopes to avoid double-weightedness, one needs to comprehend *yin* and *yang* and understand the *taiji* state.

The subsequent sentence is also very important. Wang states, "Sticking is moving, moving is sticking," which means that without there being any intent to stick to one's opponent, when one's opponent moves, one remains merged with him or her. What is called sticking requires an empty mind. If one intentionally sticks, then one's body will become rigid, while if one intentionally moves, one's body will "deflate."

Sticking and moving can be spoken of separately, but Wang reminds us, "sticking is moving and moving is sticking." When sticking and moving are spoken of at once, using a single word, this word is "transforming." Transforming must take place in such a manner that *yang* does not separate from *yin* and *yin* does not separate from *yang*—only when *yin* and *yang* mutually feed into one another can one be said to have cognized strength.

The above passage is profoundly rich in meaning; it is here where one can see why the *Treatise on Taijiquan* can simply be called "the *Treatise!*" Wang Zongyue wishes us to know that when one practices *taijiquan*, the part of oneself that is *yin* cannot exist in isolation, nor can the part of oneself that is *yang* exist on its own. *Yin* and *yang* must both simultaneously exist within a single *wuji* state.[62] The state in which *yin* and *yang* can transform into one another and mutually benefit one another is called "*yin* and *yang* nurturing one another."

---

[62] In conversation Ren elaborated on this sentence by saying, "*Taiji* has to be established upon a foundation of *wuji* in order to take form. Without *wuji*, it is impossible for there to be *taiji*. Yet the two of them exist simultaneously; it is not that first there was *wuji*, and only afterwards came *taiji*."

Anybody who can embody this philosophical principle in actual practice has cognized strength.

> "After you comprehend strength, then the more you train, the more you refine your skill. Silently contemplating and analyzing, eventually you are able to do as your heart wishes. The foundation lies in giving up the self and following others. The common mistake is giving up the close and seeking the distant. That is called 'a miniscule miscalculation that causes you to miss by a thousand miles.'"

The first two sentences above mean that as one carefully polishes one's *taijiquan*, it will become more and more refined, and eventually one's body will do just as one's mind wishes, so that in combat one feels utterly at ease.

"The foundation lies in giving up the self and following others. The common mistake is giving up the close and seeking the distant" refers to the mistake of trying to think of a way to uproot an opponent who has just made contact without first transforming his or her strength. Lots of people fight like this. If one hopes to eliminate this erroneous habit, one must learn to transform an opponent's strength from the very first moment of contact. This is the only way to be capable of moving freely. If one tries to move before having fully transformed an opponent's strength, the result is both people locking together and becoming the equivalent of a sturdy, four-legged wooden table. And, just as with a table's legs, the moment one combatant or the other gives in, the whole structure comes crashing down.

When Wang Zongyue says, "That is called 'a miniscule miscalculation that causes you to miss by a thousand miles,'" he is referring to the risk of misapprehending the fundamental concepts of *taiji*. If one loses sight of the fundamentals, there is no telling what direction one's training will veer off in. In the modern *taijiquan* world, lots of people are off by far more than just a few millimeters—they are so far off of the mark that they don't even know where to begin searching for the gate to *taiji*. This is a pitiful state of affairs.

I exhort all readers who practice *taijiquan* to endeavor to truly enter the gate. Don't just walk in endless circles outside of it. Far too many people spend endless amounts of time outside of this art's walls, never penetrating into its genuine applications and philosophical underpinnings. If one trains like this at the start of one's journey, later on the forms one practices will be completely unrelated to *taiji*.

I often ask people, "Why do you call that form you're practicing *taijiquan*? Do you think that performing a handful of moves with names like *peng*, *lü*, and *an* is *taijiquan*? If anybody could mimic those moves, why is there anything special about being a *taijiquan* practitioner?" Furthermore, when a lot of people push hands they end up just using brute strength to push back and forth. Is this infused with the spirit of *taijiquan*? Not at all! Yet large numbers of people insist upon calling this stuff *taijiquan*, which is not the least bit helpful for anybody sincerely committed to the art. Naturally, not everybody needs to become a towering master like Zhang Sanfeng, Wang Zongyue, or Yang Chengfu, but we should still expect everybody who trains this martial art to at least be walking on the correct path. At the very least, people should be able to use their training to experience what it's like to embody the philosophy of *taiji* in practice. They should be able to receive sustenance from this exquisite facet of classical culture. That is the most important thing, as it will nourish a practitioner in terms of body, heart, and mind.

> "Students cannot but be finely discerning!
> Such are my opinions."

Sincerity and compassion led Wang Zongyue to share these precious principles in writing in the *Treatise on Taijiquan*. We should be deeply grateful to our predecessors for the spirit of selflessness that led them to put the principles of the martial arts on paper as they sought to help us avoid making mistakes. Today, how many teachers and students of *taijiquan* understand why the *Treatise* is a canonical work? How many use such writings as the standard by which they measure their own martial arts training? Scarce few practitioners do so, so there is much room for improvement in our community. Wang Zongyue deserves the respect of all of us who practice *taijiquan*, and it is my deep hope that none of us will turn our backs on the theories in the *Treatise on Taijiquan* and run off to invent our own sets of ideas.

# 4

# Dispelling Doubts

*From Master Ren's discussions with students and readers*

What are the "sixteen essentials?"
What does the "tender three-inch sprout" allude to?

The sixteen essentials[63] are: agility of the waist;[64] sprightliness of the head;[65] awareness of the back; not having *qi* move to the head; strid-

---

[63] The "Sixteen Essentials" (十六關要) are emphasized by some *taijiquan* teachers, but when I asked for details about them in conversation, Master Ren said that the only reason he discusses these sixteen points is that so many students think they are important. He said he never brings them up on his own, because they were not written by Wang Zongyue and he believes they are not of great importance and not actually necessary to master *taijiquan*. He specifically asked me *not* to worry about finding a perfect way to translate or explain these terms, in order to prevent the book from losing its focus.

[64] In person, Ren added: "The agility of the body as a whole comes from being able to issue the body's movements from the waist. Moving the body with agility cannot be accomplished by trying to independently control the movements of the hands and feet, as independent movements create chaos in practice."

[65] Again, from our discussion: "A person's feelings and sensations and agility are whole-body, so the mind maintains clarity and responsiveness that allows the whole body to very quickly react. Visibly this may appear as the fighter not needing to pull his or her head down like a boxer. A stereotypical

ing with the legs; following with the feet; moving with the palms; gathering in the marrow; connecting to the *shen*; leaping with the knees; breathing with the nose; in and out breaths coming through the mouth;[66] concentrating with the ears; even distribution throughout the whole body; and expulsion through each pore on the body.

Having the "tender three-inch sprout"[67] means that by moving your entire body from your waist you gradually discover that you've created an area that can direct the agile motion of the body as a whole. This area is located just below the *mingmen*.[68] If you can truly accomplish this, then you have mastery of the internal martial arts in your future.

Recently, while practicing *taijiquan*, when I rotate the point in my lumbar vertebra it is a bit like the feeling of reeling silk from cocoons, but I don't know if that is correct or not. While training I need to constantly pay attention to this area, because as soon as I fail to do so, then it's as though it disappears. Is that how it is in the beginning? When transitioning from *peng* to *lü* while practicing "grasping the magpie's tail," should I settle my weight firmly into my

---

crouched fighting stance shows there is reactive agility in the body, whereas a *taijiquan* fighter who is totally erect in his or her stance demonstrates total, full body relaxedness."

[66] These two lines seem contradictory. Ren explained that sometimes one must use the mouth to breathe when expelling strength.

[67] This is a very literal translation of the Chinese term "三寸嫩芽." Master Ren offered the following elaboration during one of my visits to Shanghai: "When first training in using the waist to control the body, there will be the feeling that one can control the body from within the waist area. However, as *gongfu* increases, this feeling of control will extend to the rest of the body, first to the chest and then later to the head. Having a center of control in the body is like the development of a central line. The 'tender three-inch sprout' is a sensation, not an actual thing." In other words, the way of moving that Master Ren teaches begins in the *mingmen* region like a "sprout" emerging from a seed, and grows out from that region to encompass the entire body.

[68] A footnote explaining the *mingmen* can be found in He Jihong's foreword.

front leg, or should it already be settled into my hind leg? Finally, when I am straining to straighten my waist I seem to clench my teeth. How can I avoid doing so? Thank you!

At this stage, the lumbar area should feel as though it is lifting your entire body into space, and at no time should you let that feeling slip away. While training *taijiquan*, regardless of whether you are in a bow stance or a cat stance,[69] if you let your weight settle solidly down into your legs, then that is a sign that your waist has lost its strength. How can you move with agility if you settle your weight into your legs? While straightening your waist, the straightening should be done in a subtle, agile way. Do not exert too much effort while straightening your waist. Clenching your teeth is probably a symptom of trying too hard.

Photos taken of Yang Chengfu when he was young and still in the learning stage are extremely valuable, because most martial artists don't release photos of their training before they achieved mastery to the public. Clues about his manner of training are quite obvious in these photos, in which his physical posture is obviously tall and straight. The key to real skill is to gradually find relaxation and opening within tallness and straightness. One definitely should not try to relax with a shrunken little posture. Take a close look at how Yang Chengfu stands with his waist drawn upwards like a confident general surveying a battlefield. All of these points are things that beginners need to pay attention to.

---

[69] In the former stance, the majority of one's weight is on the front leg; in the latter stance, the majority of the weight is on one's back leg. The latter stance is also sometimes called an "empty stance," because the front leg is barely carrying any weight.

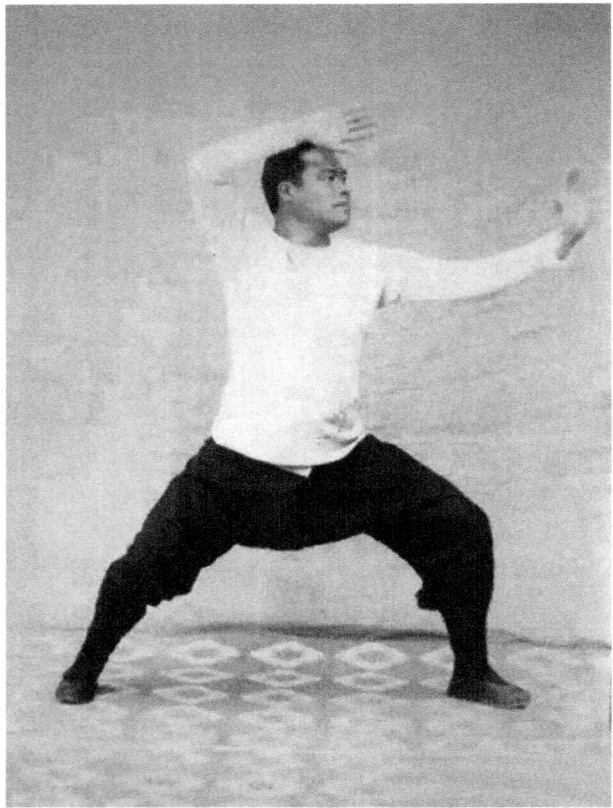

Yang Chengfu

Please explain "concentration at the crown."[70]

Having *qi* concentrated at the top of your head reflects improper training that has led the lower half of your body to become stiff and the upper half of your body to become energetically congested. It is the exact opposite of being light and agile. Dizziness and headaches are symptomatic of this condition.

---

[70] The student is asking about a term, "聚於頂," which refers to what Master Ren discusses below.

What does it mean to "leap from the knees?"

This means that once you have stored up force, when you release strength your knees should move in tandem under the control of your waist.⁷¹ Remember: this definitely does *not* refer to having the waist moving under the control of your knees!

You teach that the waist should lift and soften the whole body, and you also teach to sink the pelvis (photos of Yang Chengfu doing martial arts show him like this). Aren't those two instructions contradictory? If the waist is lifting and softening the entire body, then strength should be exerted upwards. If the pelvis is sunk, then strength should be exerted downwards. How should one deal with this when training? Also, I still haven't figured out how to straighten my waist. This morning when I was training *taijiquan*, when I reached a certain movement in the form, my teacher had me stand still and straighten my waist. He then lightly pushed me from behind and I toppled over. He shook his head and said I'm straightening my waist incorrectly, and that instead of having my waist be lifted forwards, the *mingmen* area of the lower back should be rounded outwards. I really can't figure out exactly how you're supposed to lift the waist. Also, why was I unstable when I was standing and he pushed me?

---

⁷¹ To "store force" (蓄勢) is to store up energy, while "releasing strength" (放勁) means to expel it outwards. Concentration of energy comes first, and expulsion of energy comes second. Master Ren asked me not to worry too much about translating these terms with extreme precision, because even precise wording is effectively imprecise in the eyes of a reader who lacks direct experience, while those with direct experience will easily detect Ren's point even if the wording is imperfect. With regards the relationship between the words "energy" (能量) and "Qi/qi" (炁/氣), he said: "If there is sufficient energy, we call this Qi; if Qi is sufficient to influence the external world, then we call it *shen*." As for "strength" (勁), it refers to "the practitioner's body coordinating with the energy in such a way as is capable of creating all manner of tangible effects."

If you don't straighten your waist, then it's impossible to relax your pelvis. Only when the waist is uplifted while the pelvis sinks downwards will the area between them be relaxed and open. Otherwise the waist will be restricted and lose its centeredness.

When straightening the waist it should first go forwards. Once you are skilled with this, then uplift your waist like Yang Chengfu does in his old photos.[72]

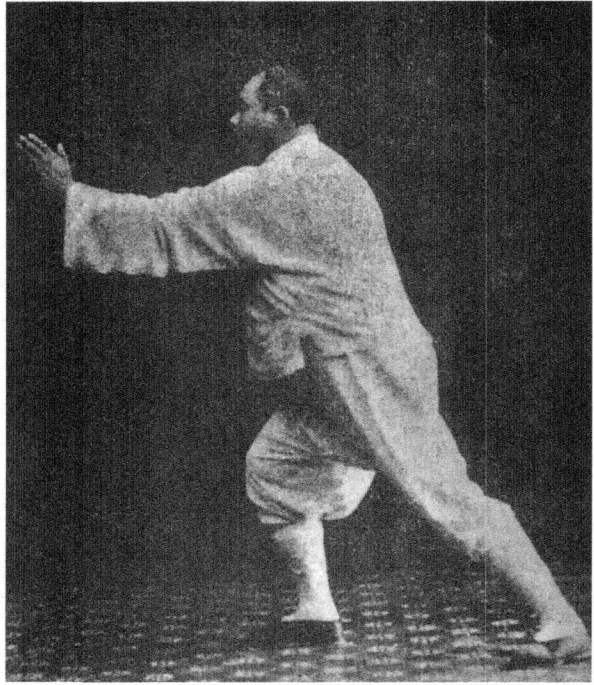

Yang Chengfu

---

[72] Ren Gang elaborated to me that since most people have a lifelong habit of letting their lower backs slump, they must first develop the physical habit of straightening their waists. After establishing this *physical* habit, they can then establish an internal, energetic habit of "uplifting" the waist, and thereby the rest of the body. It is very hard to describe this feeling in words, but Master Ren suggested that readers who really wish to know should go stand half-submerged in water at the beach or in a river and then pay attention to how the body naturally "lifts from the waist" when one is controlling one's movements while standing on an uneven surface.

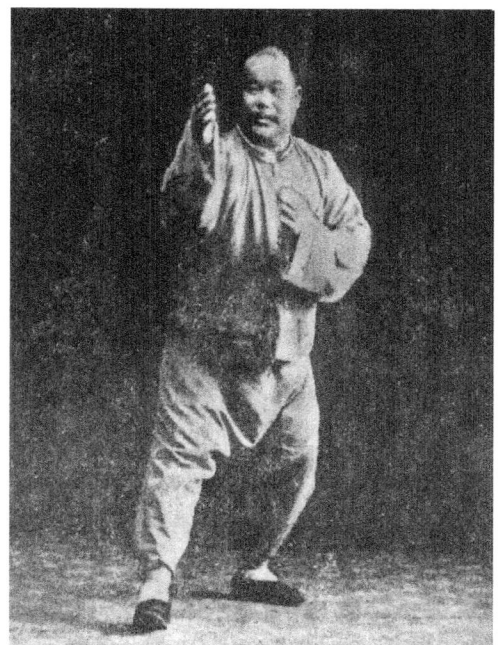

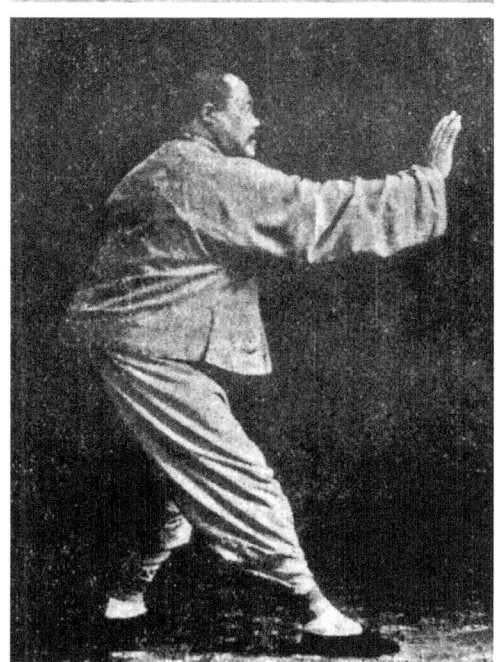

Yang Chengfu

There are a lot of people who teach that the lumbar should be rounded backwards, but I don't know what they base this idea on. I believe this is a mistake that has misled countless practitioners.

There is a *taijiquan* teaching which states that before and after one has developed a "true waist,"[73] one needs to lift the palms and sink the wrists to make them into a fulcrum for the exertion of strength. How do you interpret this statement?

Before you have developed a "true waist"—or, if you have already developed a true waist but you still haven't fully developed your strength—you can't yet totally rely upon your waist to connect with the rest of your body. You will need to use lifting your palms and sinking your wrists to assist with relaxing and opening your whole body while performing the movement *an*.[74] However, once your waist's strength is sufficient, then you need to relax and expand your palms. Once you have the true waist, if you cannot relax and expand your palms, then that is a problem.

Master Ren, I've already trained for about a month using your methods. I feel that the strength in my waist is already sufficient, and I can lift and relax my entire body without lifting my palms and sinking my wrists. This might be because I've already trained *taijiquan* for more than a decade. Now, when I lift up a point in my lumbar vertebrae, I feel that below my *mingmen* everything is relaxed, hanging, and soft. Above, my chest and arms are also very soft and open. While pushing hands, because I'm using this point in my lumbar to go forwards and backwards as well as rotate, it feels like my strength

---

[73] Ren told me that the "true waist" (真腰) is a term indicating that one is able to uplift and control the whole body from the waist, reacting instantaneously to sensations. It is a reference to a sensation of bodily control, not a discrete feeling in the lumbar region.

[74] "按" is one of the uses of force in *taijiquan*.

has grown significantly. Additionally, I feel enormous—if the person I'm pushing hands with has skills that are inferior to mine, then I feel a bit like a grown up bullying a child. Is what I'm describing correct? I still think that I have yet to develop a "true waist." Once I do, will I become even more formidable?

Also, a certain essay on *taijiquan* reads, "As for the waist's gradual development, it should extend down to the ankles... Therefore, one should use the heels instead of the palms as one's fulcrum." I'd like to ask two questions. One, how should one understand the instruction to use the heels as a fulcrum? Two, should I continue to lift my palms and sink my wrists for now, and wait until I can use my heels as a fulcrum before relaxing my palms? Or should I start relaxing my palms now?

What you describe seems to be more or less correct. When the "true waist" is first being cultivated it starts out below the *mingmen*. At this point the entirety of the waist below the *mingmen* is straight and free from the pelvis' control. Once you have created the true waist then your power will be formidable—the correct feeling is akin to being a hero on the battlefield mowing through enemies like they were grass.

If your waist's strength is fully developed then you should not lift your palms, but fully developing the waist's strength is extremely difficult. Do not think succeeding at this is a simple matter.

Regarding using the heels as a fulcrum, when you get to this point it will feel like your body is standing on emptiness, much as Master Hao Weizhen meant when he wrote, "Your feet are standing upon the surface of water."[75] At this time, each and every part of your body will be able to act as a fulcrum, with an ease and agility that is seldom seen.

---

[75] From "脚踏水面之境."

Master Ren, when speaking about *zhanzhuang* you once said,[76] "The correct training method is to first relax and expand whole body strength, and then the *mingmen* area on your back should be very subtly lifted upwards. Use this lifting strength in your lumbar to relax and expand your entire body. Relaxing and expanding is different from slack relaxation." What I would like to ask is, why should we "first relax and expand our whole body strength?" If we expand our strength, won't that make us tense? Can you explain how to expand strength?

Also, is it the entirety of the waist that lifts the whole body, or a single point upon the waist that does so, or perhaps the lumbar vertebrae? I am new to *taijiquan* practice, so these questions are really important to me. Please explain in detail.

It's quite easy for the average practitioner of *taijiquan* to confuse relaxation with flaccidity. Only after one's soft tissues and bones have been pulled into openness is it possible for there to be internal relaxation and expansion as well as circulation of *qi*. Conversely, in a state of flaccidity there is no *qi* circulation. Moreover, one cannot cultivate intuitive responsiveness on the basis of flaccid softness.

As for lifting the waist, start with the vertebra at the *mingmen*.[77] Relaxation is the state that comes when you make your interior open and connected while your strength pulls and expands. There is definitely no contradiction.

---

[76] *Zhanzhuang*, from "站樁," is sometimes translated as "standing like a post." It is a blanket term for static standing postures used in Chinese martial arts, *qigong*, and Daoist cultivation. *Zhanzhuang* practices range from the very low stances employed in Shaolin martial arts to easy, high stances that are more commonly used for *qigong* or meditation purposes.

[77] I sought clarity on this point with Master Ren in person, and he told me that practitioners should *not* worry about finding a precise anatomical location for the *mingmen* and the lumbar vertebra. A general, almost vague feeling of the area is all that is needed to train properly. He also emphasized that one starts training with the segment of the back just *below* the *mingmen*. This is because if one begins training too high of an area on the waist, then the legs are not in the scope of one's control and the body will tend to slump.

Use straightening the waist and uplifting the waist to gradually open and connect those parts of your physical interior which are not open and connected. Remember: relaxation means upliftedness. It never means floppiness.

I consistently have freezing cold toes while I'm training *taijiquan*, especially when the weather is chilly. They stay that way even after I finish training. What causes this?

Experiencing cold toes during training is caused by having a cold physical constitution. When there is an excess of cold *qi* in one's body these sorts of phenomena arise during training. Some people's feet go cold, while for others it may be their hands. You will need to stop drinking cold beverages and eating foods with cold *qi* like crab. You will also need to increase the amount of martial arts training you do, as you need to get your body to sweat profusely. Additionally, the placement of your legs and your waist in your stance is incorrect, and the stiffness in your shoulders and chest is quite obvious. Use your waist to uplift and relax these places where you have a habit of using stiff strength. Using your waist in this way will make you have an internal sensation of relaxedness and movement. Your entire body will then gradually transform into a state of openness. Only once that has happened is it possible to start contemplating having unified strength and a unified body.

Also, do not remain attached to eating crab and other seafood, because if you fail to expel the cold *qi* from your body then later on you will suffer from rheumatic disorders. When I was a student, my teacher required all of us eliminate cold foods from our diet, in addition to abstaining from tobacco and alcohol.

Master Ren, there are two methods in *taijiquan*, "touching" and "sticking." I have gleaned a few insights with regard to sticking. Namely, when touching hands with an opponent, one should have one's waist adhere to the opponent's center of gravity. One then follows along with the opponent's use of strength, rotating and folding, in order to take away his or her root. Once this is done, then both pulling in and repulsing the opponent become easy. However, I remain befuddled when it comes to "touching." What's the essential difference between touching and sticking, and how should they be applied when pushing hands? I look forward to receiving your pointers!

"Touching" refers to guiding—it is a method. "Sticking" means providing impetus—it is internal strength. Both of these are forces, not specific hand-to-hand techniques.[78]

Master Ren, can you explain to us what the masters of old meant when they referred to having ample strength in the waist?

---

[78] Above, "touching" is "沾," "sticking" is "粘," and "folding" is "摺叠." The above discussion is hard to picture, so I asked Ren for more details in person. He said, "When using *taijiquan*, if an opponent can neither shake me off nor resist me, I have 'touched' him or her. As for 'sticking,' in push hands this means I go along with feelings, following the flow of force without resisting or losing my connection. 'Folding' refers to the fact that when one wants to increase the amount of force one is using, there must be an overlap." Master Ren then demonstrated how, for example, if I were attacking him, then he would 'touch,' and no matter how I advanced upon him he moved right along with me. This created a situation in which I dared not break the connection, because then I would be open to attack. He used 'sticking' in the opposite way. While I tried to retreat he remained stuck to me, automatically following my movements. For the same reason as above, I dared not try to break the connection. A 'fold' is what allowed Ren to go from the above two relatively neutral techniques to taking the upper hand outright. While continuing to use touching/sticking, he added a directional switch to his whole-body movement, so that he was both following along with me while also moving into the opposite direction as soon as the opportunity presented itself. Doing so allowed him to advance offensively with tremendous power. The shape of the path that force takes in a "fold" is a bit like an S, in that it comes back around, both following force and taking advantage of it.

There is actually no upper limit when it comes to what counts as ample strength in the waist. The minimum standard is having no place in your entire body that is not under the guidance and control of your waist. For strength to be considered ample, neither effort nor focused attention should be necessary for you issue control from your waist. At this stage, as soon as your mind moves, the entirety of your body from head to toe—right down to very miniscule parts of your body—will naturally move with your mind. Old masters called that "not even knowing how your hands dance and your feet leap."

Master Ren, when it comes to "uplifting the waist," what are the requirements for the *mingmen* and for the tailbone? Also, how should lifting the waist affect the perineum? Should the *mingmen* be as though very slightly indented? How should the tailbone and perineum be placed? Should the crown of my head, my perineum, and the heels of my feet be in a single line, or should it be the crown of my head, my tailbone, and my heels in a single line? Should my *mingmen* area also be included along one of these lines?

The only requirement for lifting the waist is having your entire body be both uplifted and relaxed. Don't try to manage so many different things. Once you have developed the "true waist," then gradually the line of connection from head to toe will come about very naturally. It is not something that can be achieved through the intentional placement of your body parts.

I would like to ask, what does it mean to have a constitutionally cold body? Where does cold *qi* come from? Which foods count as having cold characteristics? I lived in Shanghai for several years but I never ate any of the popular crab dishes. I do, however, enjoy drinking tea. Does tea have a cold character?

There are two types of cold constitutions: innately cold body types, and those brought about by acquired lifestyle habits. The main cold foods are crab and persimmons. Some tea is cold in character. You will definitely need to train *taijiquan* in such a way that causes you to sweat profusely in order to overcome this. Cold *qi* will only be expelled from the body once true *qi* has been activated.[79] Other types of exercise which don't activate true *qi* are not ideal when it comes to dealing with cold *qi*. In the early stages of your martial arts training you should endeavor to practice outdoors, assume lower standing stances, and really get moving. You cannot cut any corners in *gongfu*.

**Master Ren, how long should it take to practice the long form? It usually takes me about 50 minutes each time.**

The length of time one spends training should be decided naturally—there's no need to set rigid goalposts. In the early stage when their movements are quite messy people tend to train the form fairly quickly. Later, when people understand what the form should ideally look like but their bodies cannot yet produce the desired effect, their training will slow down. After body and mind have been tempered by long-term training, once again the form can be trained fairly quickly. Each of us is at different stages, so there's no need to be forceful in our pursuits.

---

[79] True *qi*, from "真氣," is closely related to the terms "*Qi*" and "primordial *qi*" that Master Ren has already used. This word is often used in Daoist inner alchemy texts to refer to *Qi* after it has been made active within the human body through cultivation practice. While *Qi* is always and everywhere present, to the unachieved individual it does no more than sustain life. Conversely, when active in the body, *Qi* is understood to often promote deep-level healing and transformation via true *qi*. Even though the activity of true *qi* is determined by *Qi*, the apparent (true *qi*) the fundamental (*Qi*) are not entirely the same thing. Please note that in Chinese medicine, true *qi* is closer in meaning to "rightening/correct *qi*" (正氣).

In terms of what is required of the legs, what exactly are the limits when it comes to practicing forms with low stances? Should one assume a posture like Master Li Yaxuan's?

Without abandoning the principle that your waist should always be capable of directing the movements of your whole body, you should try to stand as low as you can. In *taijiquan* training, strength and whole-body integration need to be simultaneously cultivated. This means that once you succeed at being able to have your waist evenly uplift your entire body so that it feels empty, you should then lower your stance until the point that whole-body integratedness breaks down. From there, start your training of even integratedness anew.

Master Li Yaxuan was a practitioner of Yang style *taijiquan* who really and truly grasped the essence. It would be impossible to train like him right from the start, so one has to arrive there step by step. However, be careful not to lower your standards as you seek to lower your stance. You must keep your pelvis open and rounded. The groin area must not be drawn to a narrow angle.

I have read Li Yaxuan's books *Notes on Taijiquan* and *A Discussion of Taijiquan*.[80] Master Li describes the ways of relaxing in each and every chapter, and especially emphasizes mental relaxation. He describes total relaxation and softness, which seems to me as an instruction that is not wholly appropriate for beginners, and rather is suitable for those who already have a certain level of proficiency. At high levels, in the state in which *shen* and *qi* are extraordinarily sensitive, there can be no tension. While that state is extremely difficult to express in words and my disagreement may appear like a semantic quibble, I think that Li's choice of the words "relaxation" and "softness" may lead to misconceptions about the high-level state of "no tension." This is why I recommend regularly studying the photographs taken of predecessors like Yang Chengfu and Li Yaxuan instead of relying solely on writings about *taijiquan*.

---

[80] 《太極拳隨筆》 (*Tai Ji Quan Sui Bi*) and 《談太極拳》 (*Tan Tai Ji Quan*).

Master Ren, could you please briefly introduce the methods of *zhanzhuang*?

Just as with the practice of *taijiquan* forms, in *zhanzhuang* you should straighten the lumbar, open the pelvis, round out the angle formed in the groin where the thighs meet the trunk, and relax your whole body by subtly raising it upwards. Once you reach proficiency with these points, then continue to train with them while you are in motion. When these points no longer elude you while you're in movement, then you're practicing the *taijiquan* form properly. *Zhanzhuang* is an excellent method for speeding up the development of skill and power.

I have trouble with *zhanzhuang*. When I try to stand in a *zhanzhuang* posture, my center of gravity is essentially in my heels, whereas the fronts of my feet remain empty. However, I have heard that in *zhanzhuang* training one's toes should grip the ground and *qi* should be connected to the *yongquan* points.[81] I really don't understand what that means.

Your line of questioning suggests that your waist is still incapable of directing the movements of your entire body. Once you have trained to the point that it is as though your feet grew directly from your waist, then you will feel as though you are standing upon emptiness and your feet only very subtly touch the ground.

I have three questions. One, while training *taijiquan* or *zhanzhuang*, what should I do if a place on my body becomes very itchy? Should I take a break to scratch it? If I don't then it can become unbearable and then I can't focus my mind. Two, when I complete a *taijiquan*

---

[81] Written as "湧泉," this is the first acupuncture point on the kidney meridian. It is located on the sole of the foot and is sometimes called "Kidney 1" or "K1" in English texts on Chinese medicine

practice session, should my breath still be as even as it would be if I hadn't just been training? If I'm noticeably out of breath, does that indicate that I've somehow been training incorrectly? Three, what is the optimal speed for practicing *taiji*? When I first start the form I can go quite slowly, but the further along I get the faster my movements become, almost as though they're out of my control.

One, if you have an itch, scratch it. Two, when you have finished training the form your breath should be deeper and slower than before you started. You shouldn't be out of breath. Three, the appropriate pace for training the form is different for different levels of skill, which I already explained above. Just be natural.

There is an idea in *taijiquan* literature along the lines of, "With advancing and retreating there must be transformation; with leaving and returning there must be folding." Do "transformation" and "folding" here refer to the same thing? I have a fairly clear idea of what folding refers to, but I'm quite unsure what transformation means. I eagerly await your explanation.

"Transformation" in the context of advancing means that you move with the accumulated power of an ocean wave, while in the context of retreating it means you return like a wave that, having beaten onto the shore, takes objects on the shore back into the ocean with it. "Folding" implies that when approaching or retreating you cannot go in straight lines. You can only create force if you fold and rotate.[82]

May I ask whether there are particular instructions regarding the shoulders in the *taiji-hunyuan* standing posture? What are they?

---

[82] In conversation Master Ren told me that "folding" and "rotating" ("摺叠" and "旋轉") are one and the same action. Or, put another way, when creating force, folding cannot be executed in absence of rotation, and vice versa.

I apologize, I have never trained this type of *zhanzhuang* and I'm not privy to its details. That said, while the standing postures in *taijiquan* vary from one style to another, their underlying principles are generally the same. There should be no harm in training this posture using the principles laid out in this book.

Master Ren, I would like to ask you to explain an idea in a piece of writing on the sixteen essentials of *taijiquan* which reads, "You breathe through your nose, while the in and out breaths go through the mouth." What does that mean? I'm aware that students should not haphazardly attempt to train the inner teachings of *taijiquan* before their training has reached a certain level, so I'm just hoping to understand the principles.

Also, the best way to nourish the *shen* is to have a clear mind and not harbor too many desires. You have also suggested going to sleep before 11pm, but that seems to preclude the ancient advice that 3 to 5am is the best time to train. How can these things be reconciled?

Lastly, having seen your responses to questions people asked online about noises coming from the joints during practice, my guess is that you reached a high level in your training while you were still a teenager, and that there haven't been any breaks in your training since then. I believe that cracking noises in the joints mainly occur for practitioners who don't have enough *qi* to fill up and nourish the spaces between their bones. As long as they persist in training the proper methods while taking care of their *shen* and *qi*, then typically no serious problems will arise. Am I right?

Physical breathing takes place through the nose and should be both deep and slow. But at the same time your mouth should relax, because nasal breathing is insufficient when you're storing and expelling force, and you need to use your mouth. If you don't use the mouth at such times it's easy for *qi* to get stuck in the chest region. With regards noises in the joints, I honestly do not know what the cause is.

The ancients recommended training between 3 and 5 o'clock in the morning because they tended to go to sleep between 7 and 9 o'clock in the evening. Why would they have gone to bed as late as we do now? Modern *taijiquan* practitioners' generally low skill level is related to going to sleep too late at night.


Master Ren, could you please discuss the so-called "opening and closing of the waist?"

In actuality, in *taijiquan* opening and closing cannot be trained on an individual part of the body. Rather, the entire body needs to open and close as one. When one's skills are highly refined, then each and every part of the body from head to toe will open and close together. At that point, if there are places that don't open and close then that means that stiff strength has yet to be transformed.[83] This is especially true if it is the lumbar that cannot open and close.

---

[83] In discussion, Ren clarified to me that "stiff strength" refers to a habitual way of using the body, not the physical stiffness of a part of the body. Wherever one still has the habit of using local muscles in an isolated manner to move a part of the body, that area is effectively disconnected and cannot coordinate with the rest of the body. Instead it will act alone. Master Ren had me stand up in order to experience this point. He first had me grab his arm while it was at his side and use my strength to try and forcefully immobilize his arm. He demonstrated how he could use his own muscular strength to move my arm out of the way. He succeeded in doing so, but it was tiring for him and caused him to tense up. He then showed me the proper usage of *taijiquan* principles by letting go of the habit of individualized usage of his arm and instead moved everything (according to Ren, "everything" included "heaven and earth"). When he did this, he smoothly and effortlessly moved me out of the way. We then tried another position, in which he held up his hand as though he was about to rain a blow down upon me, but had me grab his wrist to prevent the blow from falling. When he used his arm in isolation, he had to exert himself mightily to use muscles to bring his arm down. However, when he used whole body strength his arm slid downwards naturally. His final demonstration was what a punch would feel like when using just the muscles involved in a punch compared with using the whole

Master Ren, when I practice your methods and try to use my waist to lift myself up, it feels like the upper half of my body is sitting on my waist, but at the same time I end up with a sore lower back!

There are two problems at play here. First, when you're straightening your waist, there should still be a sense of emptiness and agility. Try hard not to stiffly straighten your back—emphasize the mental aspect and deemphasize using your musculature and skeleton. Second, soreness in the lower back is a part of the training process, and it may indicate that your lower back has a chronic injury. Once you pass out of this stage things will improve.

Today while I was training I quite purposefully relaxed my shoulders and was very surprised to find that my arms instantly became soft in the way that fluids are soft. However, there was no obvious sense of relaxation in my chest and abdomen or in my lower limbs. Could you please explain why this happened, and what I should do as I continue to practice?

What you experienced counts as a good thing. When this sort of sensation extends throughout your entire body then it means that your body is as one. Keep in mind that the fluid-like state is the key. Your state should definitely not be like that of a floppy piece of cloth.

My understanding of the *taijiquan* term "hanging the groin" is that the anal sphincter muscles should be contracted upwards. However, I find that it's very hard to use these muscles, and as soon as I lift them up forcefully I create tension. What should I do?

I am not aware of there being any such training method in *taijiquan*.

---

of the room. The difference was clear. Although he did not land a blow on me, it was clear which type of hit would be more devastating.

Can you discuss the *wuji* and *taiji* postures in *zhanzhuang* practice? Although these two postures are very simple I still find them difficult to master.

My training in *taijiquan* began with the twenty-four *zhanzhuang* postures that my master taught me, so I have never trained in these two postures. Nevertheless, the governing principles should be similar. I've already written quite a bit about these principles, so it might be a good idea to review that information.

Sometimes while I'm practicing *taijiquan* I feel a current of nearly imperceptible *qi* rising from my tailbone or the *yongquan* points on the soles of my feet all the way up to *baihui* at the top of my head.[84] When this happens I'll suddenly feel woozy, although not intensely so. Am I doing something wrong?

This situation reflects the beginning stages of the growth of *shen* and *qi*. Do not seek after it. Just let it gradually grow.

Hello! After I finish training *taijiquan* my heart rate increases but I'm definitely not out of breath. Is this as it should be?

It is! As long as your heart rate doesn't surpass 130 beats per minute then it's fine.

What is an appropriate length of time for each session of *zhanzhuang*?

---

[84] The *baihui* or "百會" point, also used in acupuncture/acupressure and emphasized in *qigong*, is located at the crown of the head.

A *zhanzhuang* session where you are using a high stance should last for thirty minutes or more. If you're using a low stance then you should stand until you can no longer hold the posture. Whether you are using a high stance or a low stance, you should have at least three sessions each day.

I have been practicing standing in a low horse stance almost daily for nearly two months. My legs have become stronger, but because I haven't thoroughly grasped all of the requirements for this stance I'm always readjusting my posture when I train. I haven't been able to surpass five minutes in a single session, but each time the experience is different. Sometimes my legs feel like they're burning, other times they shake, and other times it's my back or head that becomes hot. Sometimes I end up holding my breath, which causes me to gasp for air when I'm finished. I don't know if these are all normal reactions, or if I'm practicing *zhanzhuang* incorrectly.

The sensations you describe are all normal, except for one: holding your breath. Needing to hold your breath reflects that you are using your chest to breathe. When training *zhanzhuang* you should be breathing in a way that employs your abdomen. Never hold your breath.

When I practice *zhanzhuang* it feels as though the whole of my weight is pressing down into the area beneath my knees. My knees become stiff and the soles of my feet seem to be under such intense pressure that they go a bit numb. The result of all of this is that my knees tend to hurt the following day, and the pain still remains several days later. Recently each *zhanzhuang* session has resulted in a bout of sore knees. Can you please tell me how to overcome stiff legs and pain in the knees?

When practicing *zhanzhuang* you must wear flat-soled shoes, never shoes with a raised heel. Straighten your waist and stand as though your legs were hanging from your waist. Don't relax your body in such a way that it weighs downwards. Rather, look for the sensation of standing in space.

During *zhanzhuang* practice, should one always feel like one is bracing the groin open?

No, the instruction is to round out the angle of the groin, not to brace the groin.[85]

I've recently had a few glimmers of insight into what to do with my waist during practice, but I'm not sure if they're accurate or not, so I still feel a bit confused. I've written them down here in the hope you can give me some pointers. I apologize for the awkward wording. In my state of confusion it's very difficult to clearly describe sensations that aren't clear to begin with.

What I feel is that my waist is a bit like an electrical transductor or a Y-shaped join between three pipes, and that the movements of my limbs are controlled by the transductor that is my waist. This control isn't like the normal way people rotate their waists and legs. Rather, it's control over the direction or "afflux" of my "internal

---

[85] These instructions are somewhat difficult to convey in words, but they are discussed in more depth later on. Master Ren commented that to the untrained eye both ways of standing may appear exactly the same. A person who is bracing uses strength to intentionally push the knees apart in order to open up this angle in the body. On the other hand, rounding is done in a very natural manner. The feeling the practitioner experiences with these two different approaches is very different, even if they appear nearly identical to an observer. One sign that the groin is rounded is that, from the knees downwards, the legs are basically perpendicular to the ground. The groin's "rounding" allows the upper and lower halves of the body to connect, and lets the legs' movements derive from the *mingmen*.

movements." These "internal movements" feel somewhat like a fluid, and they always pass through my waist as they move out to my four limbs. For instance, when my weight shifts from my left leg to my right leg, the "internal movement" goes through my waist as it "flows" from left leg to right (that is a simplified description—in actuality the "inner movement" occurs simultaneously in both the left and right legs, with differences in the degree of "flux" in each leg), thereby causing the gross movement of my center of gravity from my left leg to my right. The movements of my hands and arms also occur as my waist's control over "internal movement" passes from my back up and out to my fingers. Within a single whole body movement, the motions of each individual body part are simultaneously initiated by the "internal movement" that my waist controls. This occurs without there being any breaks in the process.

I'm not clear whether or not this "internal movement" is the "internal strength" that some *taijiquan* practitioners speak about. Are my pathways of "flux" what others call the "pathways of strength?" I'm still not clear what the proper pathways for my "internal movements" and "flux" are, nor how to activate specific routes for these things to take. All I have are my ongoing experiences from training *taijiquan*. Finally, when my "internal movements" are incorrect or the pathways are incorrect, it feels like my movements are extremely forced and unsmooth. Master Ren, please point out my errors and help me improve.

Some of the sensations you describe are quite on-point. As your waist can now freely move that means you have passed beyond the limitations of the lumbar's musculoskeletal structure. Next, you should come to feel how, when your waist "breathes in and out" or "swallows down and spits up," it can power the storing up and expelling of force by your entire body.[86] There should be no turn or transfor-

---

[86] This is a potentially confusing point which I discussed with Ren in person. In this context, "breathing in," "drawing in," and "storing force" are all synonymous, as are "breathing out," "pushing out," and "expelling force." Thus, it is important to be aware that so-called "breathing in and out" (呼

mation that is not controlled and governed by your waist (the key is control and governance, not flux). Moreover, for now do not try to experience internal movements. Instead, experience the whole-body flow of your *shen* and *qi* which powers both gross movements as well as internal movements. In time you will certainly reach the level of *gongfu* known as "knowing self." To be able to train to the stage of "knowing others," you will need to understand *taiji*'s philosophical principles and be able to apply them. That said, developing the *gongfu* of "knowing yourself" must come first.

What does it mean to "move *qi* with the mind?" What does it mean to "move *qi* with *shen*?"

Also, in the phrase "lift the lumbar vertebra like a taut bow about to shoot an arrow," does this mean that there is a time when the lumbar vertebra should be lifted upwards and outwards, or should the lumbar continue to be straight and slightly tilted forwards? Or should it be lifted straight up?

Finally, in the phrase "like a screw driving into the earth the left rises while the right sinks," does "the left rises" refer to a counter-clockwise rotation? Does "the right sinks" refer to a clockwise rotation?

The way this is practiced in *taijiquan* is encapsulated in the phrases "when using the mind to move *qi*, it must be made to sink" and "when using the body to move *qi*, it must be made to smoothly follow." However, note that these sentences should be understood as discussing Qi—in other words prior heaven *shen* and *qi*—rather than the *qi* in the body that comes from the nutrients we eat. One has only truly entered into the gate of internal martial arts once one is able to use the mind to move *shen* and *qi* and thereby power the move-

---

吸) and "swallowing and spitting" (吞吐) here do *not* refer to the physical actions whose names they bear, but to movements of force in the body. This is an instance where the language of *taijiquan* must not be taken too literally!

ments of the body. To do so one must use the mind, but not thoughts. Thoughts, in essence, come from mental activity and the making of distinctions. Mind, conversely, arises directly in response to the circumstances it encounters. It is my belief that insight into this point is a vital determinant of whether or not a student will plumb taijiquan's most profound depths. This is not an easy thing to understand. [87]

The teachings on lifting the lumbar vertebra refer to a state in which the waist is providing uplift to the entire body. They do not refer to simply lifting the lumbar region.

When storing up power, rotate force clockwise. When expelling power, rotate force counterclockwise.

**What do you mean when you say that storing up power is a clockwise rotation and expelling power is a counterclockwise rotation?**

This idea becomes pertinent only after you are able to use your waist to direct the whole of your body. At that point it must become a part of your training. There is actually an S-shaped reversal inside of this movement, which makes it so that when you are storing power there

---

[87] The demonstrations that Master Ren used to show me what is meant here were interesting. The gist of what he showed me is as follows: If he and I are in combat and I advance, he moves by following the force of everything involved, which includes our bodies, the room we occupy, and the space around us. His mind unites with all of these things, and therefore his body never has anywhere to get stuck, because all of these things really move as one. It is quite a bit like a fish in the sea being moved by a power that has the ability to move the fish not only by having it swim, but also by moving the water around the fish. Water of course never gets stuck, and within water all manner of forces may freely swirl. The fish, for its part, is a master when it can take advantage of these movements of force in order to increase its own capabilities of movement. In *taijiquan*, use of these principles allows a master to uproot and throw a person without stiffening up any of his or her muscles. A *taijiquan* master is always following along with the forces relevant to his or her opponent in combat. The mastery of internal martial arts comes from "merging as one with all in creation." *Taijiquan* is based on clearly distinguishing emptiness and substantiality.

is a thunderous opening up; thus, once your opponent stumbles into emptiness, your power is fully stored. After the S-shaped reversal, counter-clockwise spinning *shen* and *qi* meet one another and merge. Merged power is far greater than unmerged power.

Once this skill has been mastered, the process I just described gradually fades into formlessness. It remains present in formlessness, however, where it is none other than the basis for being able to expel power the moment you are touched.

Frequently when I'm training I'm pouring with sweat, and yet I don't feel tired. Is this abnormal? Master Ren, please let me know!

I used to be like this. I don't think there's any problem.

Can you please speak a bit about the relationship of the *dantian* to the waist in *taijiquan* training?

The relationship between the waist and the *dantian* is akin to the relationship between a commander and subordinates. If one has not cultivated the *dantian* then it is difficult to accomplish oneself, as the *dantian* is the foundation for transforming *shen* and qi. Conversely, if one has cultivated the *dantian* but not the waist, then one is like a toddler who's been let loose with a hammer.

It can also be said that successfully developing the waist is like lighting the fire beneath a cauldron. This is because the waist is a key link in the process of transmuting *jing* into qi. Cultivating a *dantian* whose contents are incapable of being transmuted into prior heaven *shen* and qi does no more than fruitlessly increase the quantities of that which desires to be spilled.

When training *taijiquan*, should one first place one's attention upon the *dantian*, and then later upon the waist?

One starts by training with the waist, because only after the waist is developed will the *dantian* be able to transform *shen* and *qi*. The contents of a full *dantian* in one who has not yet cultivated the waist are very difficult to sublimate and therefore easily cause excessive nocturnal emissions. If one cultivates one's waist and then afterwards one's *dantian*, one will wield strength as though it were a weapon forged from steel hammered a thousand times over. This is because with a properly trained waist, one is able to directly cultivate *qi* without any risks, and thus *qi* can become both vast and powerful. One's musculoskeletal system should be trained at the same time as one's waist and *dantian*. In training the physique, one should start being relaxed and extremely soft, and then become adamantine. This way, the body's interior as well as its exterior will both possess unstoppable power. In both *qi* training and physical training, the waist must act as the body's standard-bearer.

Master Ren, I would like to ask, is the idea from *taijiquan* to "gather *qi* into the bones" similar to the Buddhist white skeleton meditation practice?

"Gathering *qi* into the bones" is not the same as Buddhism's white skeleton meditation. Gathering *qi* in the bones does not imply literally gathering something in the bones on the material level. It actually means elevating the mind. Specifically this means that when you encounter an opponent's strength, you use your mind (which does not refer to the stream of thoughts in your brain) to "listen" to his or her strength. You do this in pursuit of the goal of having your body transform into an appendage of your mind.

The Buddhist white skeleton meditation is an expedient method that employs visualization in order to help people who have excessive sexual appetites. It acts as a powerful antidote to the force of habit. This method is of an entirely different nature from methods designed for worldly aims.

When it comes to Buddhist sutras that explain the distinction between thoughts and the mind, none surpass the *Shurangama Sutra*. However, this sutra is not an easy one for people who've just encountered the Dharma to comprehend. There are some commentaries on the *Shurangama Sutra* written by highly accomplished masters—having the opportunity to read one is like stumbling upon a piece of treasure.[88]

Anyway, here's a little joke: your prospects will start looking up when you finally manage to forget this heap of bones that is your body!

Hello! Your writings have given me a lot of inspiration. I've been practicing an old Chen style *taijiquan* form that I learned from a video for three years. I've always felt that I'm missing out on something internal—perhaps what I'm missing is *shen* and *qi*. Can I train the Chen form using your methods? Should I start with *zhanzhuang*, perhaps using the primordial chaos stance? If I stand for 30 minutes each morning will I obtain results? I'm sorry for asking so many questions. Thanks for your help!

You could say that giving primacy to *shen* and *qi* is what makes the internal martial arts what they are. In the end, it does not make a tremendous difference what postures and movements you use when you train, so of course it would be fine to practice what I teach within a Chen style form. If you practice in the way that I have described, then any type of *zhanzhuang* posture is fine, but I recommend you use a middle stance or low stance.

---

[88] In the Chinese version, Master Ren specifically referenced 《楞嚴經行法釋要》 (*Leng Yan Jing Xing Fa Shi Yao*) by 程叔彪 (Cheng Shubiao). This book has not been translated into English, but the sutra itself and at least one commentary are available in English.

Greetings, Master Ren! This morning I trained in a low *zhanzhuang* stance for a while, to excellent effect. My mouth produced a lot of sweet-tasting saliva in a very short amount of time, which shows that by using a low stance it's possible to obtain results without needing to set aside a huge block of time. In other words, lowering one's stance can lower the amount of time one needs to invest each day. This is really helpful for those of us with full-time jobs, as it's perfectly practical to set aside ten minutes for *zhanzhuang* three times a day, or even four or five times a day. Those with lots of time (such as retirees) can opt for higher *zhanzhuang* stances, though increasing the height of one's stance will increase the amount of time needed to obtain results. Is my thinking on the right track?

It is!


What is the relationship between practicing the *taijiquan* form, fixed stance push hands, non-fixed stance push hands, and sparring?

When practicing fixed-stance push hands, you definitely should not be standing there making circles with your training partner's hands. *Peng, lü, ji,* and *an* still need to be carefully trained in fixed stance push hands, as these four items are the most difficult to perform without sacrificing the principles of *taijiquan*. Once you can do this, then you will naturally be able to acquit yourself in non-fixed stance push hands.

Always remember that the myriad different ways of doing things all derive from the same central principles. These principles are not something you obtain from study, and yet they must be taught to you by a teacher who thoroughly understands them. If your principles are off by even a little bit, you will go bounding off in the wrong direction. Whatever you cultivate by training the *taijiquan* forms and stances will manifest in your push hands and sparring practice. Put another way, the places where you feel awkward in push hands and sparring will have their roots in your training of the form. This is why you need a readily available teacher to guide you.

There is a phrase in *taijiquan* which states "strength is exerted from the spine, shifting from foot to foot follows the body." My interpretation is as follows: In terms of the center of applied power, strength is exerted from the spine. In terms of the vector along which power is applied, it starts with the heels, goes through the spine, and is ultimately expelled from the hands. Regarding rotating so that one faces in a different direction and alternating the position of one's feet, the weight-bearing leg follows the waist's rotation, while the empty leg follows the body's opening and closing. My question is: Does all of this mean that if one is sitting on a chair there's no way to expel power? Also, if one is midair is it impossible to expel force from the spine?

"Strength is exerted from the spine" really refers to the centerline that is capable of directing the entire body. This centerline is created by concentrating the spine's *qi*; once it has taken form it can very naturally lift and direct your entire body. It should not feel as though your body is placed atop your legs; rather it should seem as though this centerline (the waist) lifts them up. Power *rises* up from the feet—it is not *pushed* up from the feet.

When you're training *taijiquan* do not settle your weight heavily down into your legs and feet, because if you do, then as soon as you become reliant on the ground your waist will not be able to command your body. However, be careful not to uplift your waist in a way that stiffens your body. Doing this should feel a bit like swimming in water, where neither foot has anywhere to be firmly planted, and your waist naturally commands your entire body. Just by training like this, eventually you will come to treat your waist as the commander of the body's movements, and you'll feel transformability, emptiness, and sprightliness as your feet naturally follow your body.

If your mind moves but your body doesn't respond agilely, this can only be because your waist's capabilities have not yet been developed.

All of the above is truly difficult to express in words. Try your best to understand their gist, and then give these instructions a try. My hope is that you won't end up with misunderstandings, because if you can get this point right then there is plenty of hope for you to make progress in *taijiquan*. You don't want to end up practicing *taiji* for a decade and still have your combat skills be worse that what they would be if you trained traditional Chinese wrestling for a couple of years!

When can a method be called "good?" If, after you've genuinely gotten the knack of a method, you start to make progress very quickly, and you get more from practicing it half-heartedly than you would from ardently practicing another method, then it's a good method. If internal martial arts didn't have this benefit, then what use would they be? The reason you constantly pay attention to your waist is that it is the link between the upper and lower halves of your body; if your waist slips away from you, then the two halves become disconnected.

Strictly speaking, consolidating power and expelling power are one and the same; transforming and striking are also one and the same. Another way to put this is that expulsion exists within consolidation and striking exists within transformation. That is why when a master's power moves it is formless, but when a beginner's force moves it follows vectors between points. Due to the limitations of language I'm afraid it would be difficult to discuss anything deeper than that level.

A lot of people can demonstrate the ability to uproot an opponent with a strike, but they can only do so when there is a major disparity between their own and their opponents' strength. There is a phrase in *taijiquan*, "As soon as my *shen* and *qi* move, my opponent is shot away like a bullet."[89] When a practitioner can only demonstrate uprooting skill against physically weaker opponents, it is questionable whether he or she is truly capable of embodying the ideal

---

[89] In Chinese: "神氣一動，彼如彈丸而出."

described in this phrase. If a *taijiquan* practitioner has to make a major effort to uproot an opponent, and in doing so tenses his or her chest and uses strength that doesn't arise from a fully unified physique, then at best all that this person can do is deliver a forceful impact. There is a big gap between that and mastery in the internal martial arts. One of my mentors used to say, "*Taiji* relies upon the sky, not upon ground. Nobody who relies on the ground has highly refined abilities."[90] I hope everybody who reads this idea will turn it over and over in their minds.

I don't know how many readers will have seriously contemplated questions such as, *Why is it that one must uproot one's opponent? In what way does uprooting an opponent assist with the expelling of power? When opponents have been uprooted, what kind of connection do they have with the surface of the ground beneath them? How do you avoid having an opponent uproot you? If you're in the midst of being uprooted by an opponent, what then is the relationship between your root and the ground below?* All of these questions pertain to training in push hands. During push hands practice, cultivating the mind is the most important point, while cultivating the body is secondary. If training does not involve the mind, then all you have is two people mindlessly making soft circles back and forth, which is less beneficial than simply practicing *taijiquan* forms.

I suggest trying the following mental-physical exercises as you search for answers to your questions: Stand in a swimming pool in chest-deep water and try to expel strength to push over a training partner. Compare this with doing so while your back is against the wall of the pool. Also, try pulling yourself out of the pool without using the ladder. Why is that so difficult to accomplish without a

---

[90] From "太極借天，不借地.借地始終藝不高." The operative character here is "天," which is usually translated as "sky" or "heaven." I asked Ren for clarification in conversation and he said the following: "In this context this character refers to the whole of space, not just the sky. The practitioner makes use of *space* rather than the earth below his or her feet and the strength that derives from pressing the legs down into it. This character is not the 'heaven' religions speak of, nor is it simply 'the sky.'"

ladder, and so easy with one? *Taijiquan* comes from nature and from daily life—its principles derive from following the course of nature to its ultimate conclusion. Humans never cease being humans, and humans never cease to have a connection with the ground beneath them.

It is somewhat inaccurate to speak about "uprooting" in the context of repulsing an opponent in *taijiquan*. A better term would be "lifting." This is because once you've guided an opponent to the point that he or she has fallen into emptiness, when you repel him or her, there's really no longer a root left to uproot.[91] If your opponent's root is still planted and then you try to forcefully strike him or her, then you're making the mistake of pushing into resistance.

---

When I lift my waist, I very clearly feel that there is something very hot at my *mingmen* which can move according to my will. Typically, as soon as I think of it, it is there. Just as you've written, now when I practice the form I am much more light and agile. One time while training my legs suddenly felt weightless, as though they were floating as I walked. This actually gave me quite a fright, but luckily it only happened once! This is my question: I've already trained for more than eight months, and now when I train lifting the waist I often sense a wave of power spontaneously traveling up my spinal column towards the crown of my head, after which my head feels a bit foggy (but not dizzy) and quite unpleasant. Where does my problem stem from, and how might I resolve it? I humbly ask for your advice.

---

[91] I asked Ren to touch hands to demonstrate what he explains here. At the time I wrote the following: "In push hands, if Master Ren is using force, then when I want to move I already feel as though my root is lost, so he does not have to use strength or any specific techniques to try and uproot me. My root is simply gone, because I feel like I am standing in an empty space that I cannot control."

Given the situation you describe you should pay attention to the following points:
1. Your lumbar should be straight and subtly tilted forwards. It should not poke out backwards.
2. Lifting the waist should only involve the region one finger-width or so below the *mingmen* point. Lift it until your whole body feels light and agile. If you go beyond that, then you will create the undesirable effect of making your body stiff.
3. Your middle *qi* should not rise above the *tanzhong* acupoint located in the center of your chest approximately between your nipples.[92]
4. The correct sensation is that you're practically capable of walking on air. Your body should feel free and easy, your limbs should feel like clouds, your thoughts should be like a crisp autumn breeze, and your body should instantaneously follow your mind's movements. Feeling that you are losing control while your head is heavy and your feet are weightless is incorrect.

**Master Ren, can you please explain what you mean by "rely" in the context of "relying on the ground?"**

First, as a student of *taijiquan*, one needs to gain a feel for the state in which self, others, sky, and earth are all merged together. From there, one will gradually begin to experience a light agility that stems from unity with everything in creation. This type of agility is a rising that naturally contains a sense of weight and firmness. It does *not* mean first drilling oneself downwards in order to spring back upwards.

---

[92] In conversation Master Ren described "middle *qi*" (中氣) as "the *qi* that moves up and down like a valve and powers the movement of the *qi* in the extraordinary vessels." He immediately added that all of these issues naturally self-correct in anybody who trains *taijiquan* with an understanding of "the individual and all things in creation merged as one" and "*yin, yang, insubstantiality, substantiality.*"

What I have just described is the beginning of "relying on the sky instead of relying on the ground."[93]

**The S-shaped reversal you described is very difficult to convey in words, so does that mean a figure 8-shaped reversal is even harder to explain?**

The S-shaped reversal is a method for controlling *shen* and *qi* that should be introduced after a student has trained to the point where the waist governs all movements and the region just below the *mingmen* uplifts the entire body. Indeed, it may be something that can only be properly conveyed via in-person coaching, as anything one might say about it ends up being incorrect.

In fact, as soon as there is an S-shaped reversal there is also a figure 8-shaped reversal. These two are one and the same. Be very careful not to overcomplicate things when you practice *taijiquan*. If you're not yet capable of having the waist control your whole body, then attempting to execute the S-shaped reversal will amount to little more than twisting your waist. Of course you can practice that, but you won't be getting any substantial results, you'll just be whetting your palate.

**At what point is the reversal executed?**

Broadly speaking, when my opponent has fallen into emptiness, then that's when I execute a reversal.

---

[93] In discussion, Ren added, "Gradually you will feel that the world's space is full of strength and the body's strength is tiny, so you will gradually let go of the body and more and more make use of space."

Is it correct to use the heels of the feet as an axis while training *taijiquan*? Should the "four cardinal hands" of *peng*, *lü*, *ji*, and *an* be distinguished and trained in isolation?

In *taijiquan* training, the waist *must* be the body's governor. Everything else is just tools in your toolkit. The four cardinal hands should be trained together in accord with *taijiquan* principles. *Peng*, *lü*, *ji*, and *an* should all be very clearly delineated within four cardinal hands practice. This sort of training should not be like what you see when some teachers just make circles with their arms. I don't know whether to laugh or cry when I see that, but the fact is that quite often *taijiquan* lessons on video are riddled with mistakes. Your best option is to ask a legitimate teacher to teach you the four cardinal hands in person, as they are very important.

While practicing *taijiquan*, my physical sensations have been gradually becoming more distinct. I'm now able to sense the extending of my bones and sinews; I can feel something flowing up and down throughout my body; I can sense my body expanding out in all directions while also contracting around my lumbar vertebra; I feel the power that slowly rises up as a result of the soles of my feet gently touching the ground; and I can feel that when all of the intent and *qi* in my body sink down into the soles of my feet then my whole body becomes relaxed and empty. These are things I can call forth and control with my thinking, and they can transform in accord with the fluctuations of my mind. Through training *zhanzhuang* and *taijiquan* forms, bit by bit I am discovering and experiencing my body's movements, as well as the way in which my mind and thoughts are gradually merging with my body. Although this merging is still clumsy and nascent, thanks to what I described my training has surpassed the stage of simply exercising my limbs.

Achieved teachers frequently warn not to get wrapped up in one's *qi* sensations, as they are all empty illusions. They warn to never seek and chase after these things. Sometimes I feel perplexed. Practicing *taijiquan* makes people's senses more acute and lets us feel the changes going on inside of our bodies, so how could we not pay attention to these things? What is the correct approach?

Everybody's physical sensations are different. To completely ignore them would be impossible, but as soon as you chase after them you've gone astray. The best approach is to devote your attention to the fundamental principles while remaining aware that everything that you feel is just part of a process. Do not harbor an attitude that all of this is somehow special and do not pursue experiences. This way you will be better off.

Master Ren, could you please discuss how to develop accurate perception?

If you wish to develop accurate perception, then first you need to know what counts as authentic *taijiquan* and what proper practice should be like. The basis of *taijiquan* lies in the philosophical principle which states that *taiji* is born of *wuji*. Training this martial art starts with lengthening the tendons and other soft tissues of the body while opening up the skeletature, so that from head to toe one's bones and flesh are all unified. So long as the methods one uses are correct, then within two to three years one can certainly complete this stage. At that point if you counter an external force you'll have a root beneath your feet and the fulcrum where you receive this stress will be in your waist instead of in your shoulders or your chest. You will then be able to withstand very strong force within a state of relaxation. After this point you then begin to train *shen* and *qi*, using your mind to move your body. Gradually your arms, your legs, and the *shen* and *qi* of your whole body will all act as one in unison with your mind, so your *shen* and *qi* will be a sovereign of sorts, and your flesh-and-blood body will be the sovereign's loyal officials. This stage in training takes another two years or so, after which point you are really doing internal martial arts. If you use the generating and restricting principles of the five phases as you move your body and your *shen* and *qi*, then what you are doing can be called *wuxingquan*. If you use the principles of the changes in the eight trigrams, then you are training in *baguazhang*.[94]

Anybody who wishes to train *taijiquan* must first understand its philosophical principles, a requirement which includes directly experiencing what is pointed to by the concept of being one with all things. This point is exceedingly difficult to realize. Firstly, one must have traditional Chinese cultural background knowledge. Secondly, one's *shen* and *qi* must be replete. Only when these two factors come together can one directly experience that which is extremely subtle.

Additionally, a legitimate teacher to point the way is still required in order for there to be any real hope of success. If you are lucky and your insights bring you into the realm of *taijiquan*, then you will need to carefully maintain this state of being and bring it to maturity. Should you reach this stage, then no matter how strong or physically imposing your opponent may be, your mind will not give birth to any thoughts of resistance. This is because you will have reached *wuji*, where you and your opponent are as one. Within *wuji* you will be able to employ any manner of application for dealing with your opponent without causing the principle of the *wuji* to break apart. From this point onwards, you will have a foundation which allows you to begin using *taiji* principles. After you can experience *wuji* with an opponent, you will feel that whenever he or she moves, he or she creates an energetic change that destroys *wuji*. This disruption is described as emptiness and substantiality. It is also called *taiji*. It is born of *wuji* at the moment when movement leads to the splitting of *yin* and *yang*.

Once you have arrived here, then if you meticulously contemplate Wang Zongyue's *Treatise on Taijiquan* you will naturally find yourself in a new world. But I emphasize, to have an epiphany that lets you

---

[94] *Wuxingquan*, named for the five phases, is written "五行拳." It is synonymous with *xingyiquan*, which is written "形意拳." *Baguazhang*, named for the eight trigrams, is written "八卦掌." These two internal martial arts are considered to be close cousins of *taijiquan*.

realize the principle of *wuji* is not easy. Some people spend a lifetime trying and yet never find the door. There is a relationship between one's chances here and one's background knowledge in Confucian, Buddhist, and Daoist philosophy.

Master Ren, I'm a greenhorn, and I'm wondering where I should start. There are so many types of *taijiquan*, so which one should I train? Can you give me some advice so I don't end up on the wrong path?

The first steps you take in your study of *taijiquan* are especially important. You may wish to begin by doing some *zhanzhuang*, which many teachers offer instruction in. The shape of a *zhanzhuang* stance and the positioning of the hands and feet are not the most important thing. What you need to pay close attention to are the following key points:

One: A lot of people say that in *zhanzhuang* or *taijiquan* practice the entire body should be relaxed. Training like this will never create a waist that is capable of governing the whole body's movements, so eventually all that will come of it is resistive strength and shoving strength, instead of long strength and sharp strength.[95] The proper method of training *zhanzhuang* is to first open up the strength of the entire body, and then very subtly straighten up the *mingmen* area on the waist. Make use of this upward-lifting strength so that the whole body is *song*[96] and open (not relaxed and flaccid) and it feels

---

[95] The first ideal is written as "抛勁," which could be translated as "throwing strength," but Master Ren suggested I call it "long strength" instead. He described it as the type of power needed to truly send an opponent flying. The second ideal is written as "冷彈勁," which could be directly translated as "cold shooting strength." "Sharp" was also his suggestion, and he described it as the ability to attack another's body with incredibly sharp, focused power. "Short strength," a synonym for this term, appears in the next chapter.

[96] "鬆" may accurately enough be translated as "relaxation" in most contexts, with the internal martial arts being a notable exception. Because its *pinyin* transliteration has already made its way into the English-speaking *taijiquan*

as though the waist is uplifting your arms, legs, and every other part of your body. In the beginning, when your waist's strength is insufficient, you will not be able to have your entire body be open and *song*, so you will only be able to achieve this in certain parts of your body. Gradually, as your skill grows, your entire body will open and *song* one area at a time. Eventually you will be able to feel that your waist is acting as the center of control.

Two: Whether training *zhanzhuang* or *taijiquan*, you should open the angle of your groin where your thighs meet your body and round out your pelvis. You must do this while maintaining the above requirements, or else your training will result in a stiff waist and pelvis. Stiffness is incorrect. If you do not open your groin and round out your pelvis, then later on it will be difficult to achieve merged power, which means you will have much less power to draw upon to repulse an opponent.[97]

There is an instruction in *taijiquan* which says "firstly lengthen tendons, secondly nurture *qi*, thirdly comprehend power, and that is all." Master Ren, can you explain how to train like this?

There are lots of foundational practices for lengthening the tendons and other soft tissues, but it's not possible to teach them in writing. You can also succeed at this by training *taijiquan* forms with an open groin and a rounded pelvis while in the bow stance or empty stance. Nurturing *qi* is an indispensable factor in the internal martial arts, as it is the foundation for both moving *qi* with the mind as well as

---

community's vernacular, I have decided to use *"song"* in instances where Ren is clearly embarking upon a discussion distinct from relaxation in its quotidian sense.

[97] Regarding the meaning of "to repulse" (發) in *taijiquan*, Ren reminded me that this means using energy to strike a person away, which is very different from using brute strength to shove a person away. "Repulsing" means expelling energy in order to an attack an opponent. This energy or power comes from space, not from bracing one's body against the ground.

relaxing and opening the entire body. However, skill in moving *qi* with your mind has to be trained while leading an orderly lifestyle, avoiding excesses, and getting enough sleep. If you devote at least three hours a day to training, then in time you will successfully nurture your *qi*. As for cognizing strength, that is comparatively more difficult. Once your entire body is *song* and open, then first you need to directly experience the principles of being one with your opponent in *wuji*. Then you must transform *jing* into *Qi* and understand force, and next directly experience the *yin* and *yang* of *taiji* so that you can gradually cognize strength.

Is there an order when it comes to lengthening the soft tissues? Where should we begin? Thank you!

Start by opening the angle of the groin, rounding out the pelvis, and straightening the waist.[98]

Is there a relationship between nurturing *qi* and lengthening the tendons and other soft tissues? Can one lengthen the soft tissues but not nurture *qi*? Also, Master Ren, may I ask which type of *taijiquan* you practice?

---

[98] I asked Master Ren to show me what these instructions look like in practice, and he stood in a simple horse stance in such a way that his feet were slightly farther apart than the width of his shoulders, and the lower half of both of his legs (starting at his knees and going down to his feet) was directly perpendicular with the ground, instead of bowed out or knocked inwards. He then said that this happens *naturally* when the groin and pelvis are open and rounded, but it can also be done *forcefully* if one uses strength to try and pull the knees apart. The former is natural and creates as well as results from openness. The latter is not a true accomplishment and will not lead to success in *taijiquan*. To the untrained naked eye, it is difficult to see the difference between the two ways of standing, so practitioners must carefully observe their bodies and *qi* in order to ascertain how to practice according to these principles.

Lengthening the soft tissues is one of the foundations of all martial arts training. It allows musculoskeletal strength to operate smoothly while increasing a practitioner's range of motion. This training is analogous to fashioning a vessel so that you can store water—the bigger the vessel, the more water you can collect.

Nurturing *qi* is foundational to internal martial arts training. When *qi* is ample it transmutes into *shen*; only when *shen* and *qi* are both replete will you be able to transform the stiff places in the body and gradually arrive at the stage where the body is a unified whole that is controlled by the mind.

I practice Yang style *taijiquan* in an orthodox lineage. Strictly speaking, the words "Yang style" are superfluous, because after you truly comprehend its philosophy, practicing *taijiquan* simply means physically enacting *taiji* principles. Each time I do the form it is different, because all I seek is for my *shen* and *qi* to penetrate into the principles. I do not strive for sameness in my physical postures when I train. How many practitioners of "Yang style" do the form the same way? Who among them are really training "Yang style," and who among them are not?

My lineage comes from the Yang family through Dong Yingjie, Yue Huanzhi, Dong Shizuo, and Dong Bin down to me.

If one's root is in one's heels, why is the fulcrum in the waist? The waist's only function is to transmit.[99] If one's fulcrum is in one's waist, then one's power is severed, so how could it arrive in one's fingers? Your theories are nonsense!

It's quite difficult to understand these principles, and that's why most people end up training resistive power. Have you heard the term, "*Taiji* relies on the sky and not on the ground," or of the three realms:

---

[99] Regarding this person's statement Ren elaborated, "His misunderstanding is that he thinks strength comes up through the body one step at a time."

"Below the water, in the water, and above the water?"[100] Are you sure you understand these teachings?

Finally, from the very earliest stages of *taijiquan* training through to the very end, the waist is always the governor. It is never used as a transmitter.

---

[100] This idea comes from Hao Weizhen, who said that people who have just started learning *taijiquan* are as though under water, with their feet stuck in muck. After obtaining a certain degree of skill, they are as though freely moving in water. Finally, if they reach mastery, it is as though they are walking on water.

# 5

# Resolving Confusion

*From Ren Gang's written correspondence with readers*

Master Ren, can you please comment on Yang Chengfu's level of achievement?

Master Yang's *taijiquan* was at the level where it was as though he was levitating, with his feet planted in his own *shen* and *qi*. His Qi was expansive and vast and beyond what anybody has since achieved.

When beginning to learn *taijiquan*, one must constantly pay attention to the waist. One starts with the lumbar vertebra, and later slowly comes to feel that where the mind is placed there lies a centerline that is empty, numinous, and capable of changing in ways that conducts the motions of the whole body. Later still, one will feel that this centerline can change positions and that it comprises the mind and not the muscles or the skeleton. This is what Master Sun Lutang was referring to when he said "anywhere in my body can act as the fulcrum, and thus there is no limit to the ways in which I can transform."

All of this comes from first training the waist. There is no way other than this. That which comes later is not meant to be spoken of, out of concern for the possibility that some people will misinterpret the words and wander down mistaken paths.

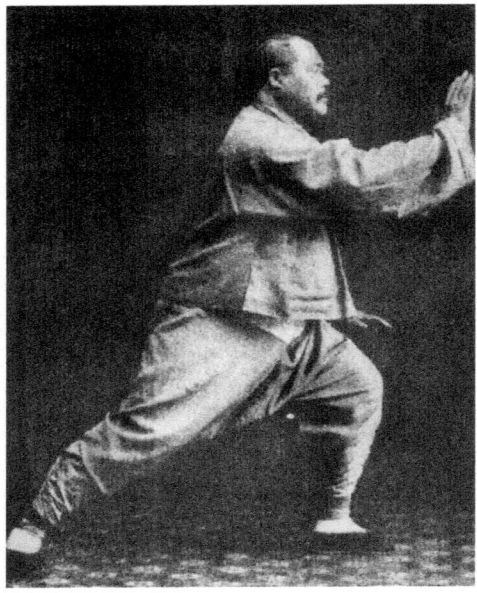

Yang Chengfu

Master Ren, what does the phrase "be not askew, be not awry; now hidden, now apparent" mean? I would very much like to hear your explanation.

"Neither askew nor awry" is very important. When you touch hands with an opponent, you should stand as though your body is the link between heaven and earth. You absolutely must not get into a situation where you and your opponent are shoving into each other, leaning on one another, or propping each other up. This way, even if your opponent suddenly vanished into thin air, you would still be standing steadily between heaven and earth.

When engaged with an opponent you also should not try to avoid or get out of your opponent's way. In *taijiquan* there is transforming, but there is no avoiding or getting out of the way. If you avoid then there will be places where your *shen* and *qi* collapse, while what you should actually aim for is to make your opponent feel as if your *shen* and *qi* are keeping them in constant, imminent peril. When an opponent places a hand on you, he or she should feel as though there is nothing to grasp onto. This will cause him or her to become deeply unnerved!

"Now hidden, now apparent" speaks to the mutability of *shen* and *qi*. What it means is that *shen* and *qi* drive the transformations of *yin* and *yang* in your body, but this is something that can only be demonstrated by a person who has an excellent foundation in the internal martial arts. It's quite impossible to portray in words.

Please would you discuss the difference between avoiding and transforming?

This is one of those questions that is exceptionally hard to address verbally. Ideally I would let you experience the difference directly, but all I can do right now is attempt to force it into words. I'm not sure if my answer will satisfy.

In "avoiding" the preponderant factors are retreating and giving way, such that *shen*, *qi*, and the body are all performing a dodge. If you do this in the face of a stronger, faster opponent then you will inevitably end up under his or her control. Thus, the ability to "avoid" is basically defined by your speed relative to your opponent's.

To "transform" means that when your opponent advances you connect to his or her force.[101] Once you have connected, regardless of whether your opponent's *shen* and *qi* continue to advance or go into retreat, you make yourself empty to dispatch with them. This will give your opponent the feeling of slipping into an abyss.[102] Perhaps the best way to explain this is that your opponent will feel that there is nothing to chase after and strike at—it is like he or she is trying to do battle with thin air.

---

[101] Master Ren elaborated to me that "connecting" (接) in this context means "joining with space, sensing the forces of the opponent's movements as well as the room around you."

[102] In person Ren said this means "forcing the opponent to lose the sensation of standing firmly and securely on even ground."

Master Ren, I have a question. If I thoroughly comprehend the *wuji* principle, will this cure my physical illnesses? I have suffered from chronic respiratory tract ailments since I was a child.

I'm very sorry, all I can say to you is that while awakening to the principles of *taiji* and *wuji* will benefit your body, curing a disease at its root level would still be very difficult.

Master Ren, early on you said that learning *taijiquan* is easy, and that people who want to succeed need do no more than find an appropriate method and apply themselves to it single-mindedly for a decade. Later you said it's very difficult, and thus most people lose the desire to keep training. Have you not contradicted yourself? Additionally, some of your insights make for useful references, but I do not agree with everything you say. For example, you said that when opponents push you, you feel their strength in your waist, but you clearly picked up this mistaken perception from the Commission for Physical Culture and Sports' standardized *taijiquan* (which mistakenly requires that the upper half of one's body be perpendicular to the ground). Well, I beg to differ. My contention is that an opponent's strength should be felt in the soles of your feet. What sayeth you?

In the study of *taijiquan* it is not difficult to understand what the proper methods and goals are. So long as a person who thoroughly understands these things explains them to you, you should be able to grasp them. However, this is simply where a path that has no endpoint begins. Nowadays people have so many hobbies and lead fairly undisciplined lifestyles, so if somebody has a dream of reaching the level of the masters of old it will indeed be quite hard to realize. Yet, be that as it may, as long as a modern person trains correctly, he or she will soon enough realize that it is possible to approach the level of our predecessors, and that if one fails to do so, then it is merely a question of not investing the requisite time and effort. People who realize this take personal responsibility for the outcome of their training, and do not blame *taijiquan* for having deceived them.

In the past people used to say: "A craftsman can only teach you the tricks of the trade—he can't give you skill itself." For example, even if Lu Ban, the master carpenter of ancient legend, wanted to teach somebody how to fashion a wooden chair, all he could do is describe and demonstrate the steps involved in making a chair. There is no way he could somehow cause a student to reach his level of exquisite carpentry overnight. In fact, in spite of having received proper instruction, even after a lifetime of practice the student still might not reach Lu Ban's level. Nevertheless, so long as the techniques Lu Ban taught the student were correct, then the student would at least be capable of building serviceable chairs.

In the early stages of your *taijiquan* training, receiving opponents' strength in your waist is not only the correct thing to do, it is also a key factor that decides whether or not you will find success in your practice of this art. Please continue to experiment with this. I have already walked this path. Why on earth would I mislead you?

If a *taijiquan* master were to face off with an enormous heavyweight boxing champion, and the boxer threw the full weight of his body into a punch aimed directly at the master's chest, is making use of the boxer's force in order to parry[103] the punch the only thing the *tai-*

---

[103] The Chinese word Master Ren used here is "腾開," which is not found in English-Chinese dictionaries as a synonym for "parry." Nevertheless, I chose parry after contemplating my conversation with Ren and the definitions of this word in *Merriam-Webster*. Ren offered extensive thoughts on this concept in person. My notes from our conversation are as follows: "'Parrying' means getting out of the way, but not in the same way of 'avoiding.' Rather, when parrying, the master still moves in oneness with force to avoid getting hit, but because he or she is still united with this force, there is no shrinking or loss in this movement, and furthermore when the parry is completed, the master is now at advantage, because he or she is still connected to force, whereas the less skilled attacker has committed to a movement using his or her body in such a way that he or she is no longer safely rooted to the ground." In response to further questioning Master Ren

*jiquan* master could do? Might the *taijiquan* master be able to merge into a single *taiji* with the boxing champion? Could the boxer's force be transformed in formlessness? Would the *taijiquan* master's legs be capable of sustaining such weight? Also, if the punch were directed towards the belly, is there a way a *taijiquan* master could transform such force? Please let me know what you think.

If you are engaged with an opponent and he or she suddenly makes a sneak attack, then you should first react by making use of your opponent's force in order to parry out of harm's way.

If you are squaring off with an opponent and, before he or she has had a chance to move, you have already harmonized so that both of you fall within the *wuji* principle, then as soon as your opponent moves, a disparity between insubstantiality and substantiality will be created. That is when you connect to your opponent's solidity, which will force him or her to fall into emptiness. Simultaneously, your *shen* and *qi* should surge into the empty spaces like lightning. The instant your body joins this movement, your opponent is guaranteed to falter.

I have crossed hands with boxers, Muay Thai fighters, aikido practitioners, and representatives of plenty of other martial arts. I can tell you that I have never lost. None of them were famous masters, but having tried my hand against these fighters I have no question in my mind as to what works and what does not.

From what you've written I have a hunch that you have seen highly skilled martial artists in action and received oral instruction from them. Don't let opportunities like that pass you by!

---

said that when a *taijiquan* master fights, force always moves first, the body second. In contrast, most fighters in most disciplines *only* move their bodies; a small number with some internal ability move their bodies first but bring force along with their physical movements (in Ren's opinion Mike Tyson is in this category, and his ability to move force with his body is part of the reason he defeated so many people). A person must learn to be one with force to master *taijiquan*. Force is found in the "place" where *yin* and *yang* can be found and separated.

Thank you for your explanation. My knowledge here is too superficial for me to claim any real understanding, so I'm hoping you can give me a few more pointers. Some people say that in *taijiquan* punches should be thrown relaxedly, but that when punches are about to land the fist should be clenched tightly. Other people say that is wrong, and that one's fist should be relaxed from start to finish because this is the only way for power to reach the hands. Also, some people say that since one uses the opponent's strength to strike in *taijiquan*, there is therefore no need to develop especially strong legs—so long as you can hold yourself up with your legs then that's enough. I'm wondering, is that similar to what you mean when you speak about relying upon the sky instead of the ground? How should this be trained?

In *taijiquan* "hardness and softness nourish one another." "Hardness" refers to *shen* and *qi* being gathered into the bones, while "softness" refers to unobstructed connectivity in the musculoskeletal structure. If your power extends into your fingers, then very naturally if you hit an opponent you will feel like he or she is no stronger than a pile of old, worn-out cotton stuffing. Your opponent will be terrified. This level of skill is what we call "*gongfu*." Once your skills are consummate, then your limbs will be both soft and weighted,[104] and a move of your hands will resemble a terrific wave crashing against cliffs. Musculoskeletal strength is simply no match for the force of *shen* and *qi*! In authentic *taijiquan*, an opponent is repulsed the moment he or she gets struck; this effect definitely does not come from power you could create by digging into the earth with your heels. In sum, there can be no stiffness anywhere if one is to use *taijiquan* to transform force and repulse an opponent. Anywhere there is stiffness a mistake is being made.

---

[104] Ren mentioned to me that this sort of "weightedness" is due to force—it is not a matter of musculoskeletal strength.

I'm a beginner who recently had the pleasure of reading one of your essays, which I gained a lot from. I am learning the Yang style old Mao Zhai form, which might be quite similar to what you practice. I say this because you emphasize "lengthening the soft tissues and opening the skeletature," which is exactly the same as one of the requirements in our form. I would like to ask you, how does one accomplish "*qi* suffusing the entire body without any blockages," and how does one determine whether or not one has done so successfully? Additionally, I would like to ask you to discuss the precise meaning of the term "lengthen the soft tissues and open the skeletature." Which famous athletes would you say have accomplished this?

It makes me very happy to hear that what I've written has been of benefit to you. Regarding "*qi* suffusing the entire body without any blockages," this is a reference to achieving the ability to control your body with mind and *qi*. Once your *shen* and *qi* are ample, then day by day, as you practice using the mind to move *qi* and using *qi* to move the body, you will sense all of the hardened parts of your body slowly softening and opening. When your whole body feels as though it is a single, uniform entity and there is no part of it that does not take part in movement, then you have more or less achieved what the phrase you asked about refers to.

*Taijiquan*'s lengthening of the soft tissues and opening of the skeletature is different from what is seen in other types of physical exercise. What *taijiquan* requires is increasing your strength while you are in a state of equipollence.[105] There are two ways of training this. In the first way, you start directly with equipollence training. Thus, in a

---

[105] Anybody who compares this text with the Chinese version will notice that equipollence ("equalness of force, power, or effectiveness") is my translation for "蕩開," "鼓蕩," and "均勻一體." This translation is not related to dictionary definitions of those Chinese terms; it is specific to conversations I had with Master Ren to clarify his terminology, as well as to demonstrations he gave me in person. Equipollence implies even, unimpeded distribution of strength and force in a person whose body is open and *song*, and whose mind occupies the *taiji* state.

small, high stance you train in such a manner as to establish whole-body equipollency, and then once you have established it you open up your stance while sitting lower on your legs until you lose the ability to remain equipollent. At that point you reestablish equipollency. This cycle is repeated as you progressively lower and expand your stance. In the second way of training, you start with an expansive, low stance at the very beginning, and you gradually train towards equipollence within this challenging posture.

Thank you for deepening my understanding of *taijiquan*. I'd like to ask, with respect to the concept of "hardness and softness nourishing each other," what did you mean when you said, "If your power extends into your fingers, then very naturally if you hit an opponent you will feel like he or she is no stronger than a pile of old, worn-out cotton stuffing. Your opponent will be terrified"? I have seen photos of people being repulsed high into the air which I believe are real, but since I personally lack this sort of power it's impossible for me to analyze what is going on. Can you explain?

When it comes to repulsing an opponent in *taijiquan*, two types of power are used, long strength and short strength. When expelling long strength, you connect to the entirety of your opponent's body, cause it to fall into emptiness, and then fling the person away as you expel your strength. Long strength can send a person flying several meters away, and yet it does not easily cause serious harm. The biggest fear is that the person receives an injury from stumbling to the ground. This sort of strength is usually employed when there is a large disparity between you and your opponent's level of skill.

When expelling short strength, you only connect to an isolated point on an opponent's body, for instance his or her heart, lungs, or liver. Your *shen* and *qi* slice inwards to attack in an instant. Although such a blow may not cause the recipient to be repelled by any significant distance, it can very easily cripple a person. When I said an opponent would be terrified, I was referring to the moment at which he or she is on the receiving end of such power, as it will cause an injury.

Unless you have total mastery over it, short power is usually reserved for martial competition or dire circumstances. In order to produce short power you must have very substantial *shen* and *qi* as well as visualization ability, and furthermore your entire body must be open and connected.

Release of energy is a major component of the strength used in *taijiquan*, which is not at all the same as simple striking power. The role of energy release in this kind of strength is related to the way a person who is electrocuted will be sent flying, whereas a block of wood will not be moved by electric shocks. That said, receiving a blow from a *taijiquan* master and electrocution are not really the same thing. Perhaps *taijiquan* is a bit like a combination of the factors at work in both simple striking power and electrocution.

How does one deal with and take advantage of gravity within the context of *taijiquan*'s postures? This is quite a broad question, and since we are communicating in writing I daren't ask you to write a terribly thorough response. I'm simply hoping you will describe one or two practicable methods. I am sure many people would reap extensive benefits.

The first thing to do is train in order to link all parts of your body into an equipollent unity that responds in its entirety the very instant your waist moves.[106] You'll only be able to work with your body's weight once you have reached this stage. When your waist can act like a sort of director general that powers the rest of the body, you're ready.

---

[106] Master Ren clarified that this complicated-sounding instruction is no different from the previous chapter's concept of there not being any areas of stiffness in the body. Recall that stiffness is not so much a physical state as "a habit of using stiff strength."

While you train each part of a *taijiquan* form, always imagine that you are engaged in an actual fight with an opponent. Each place where you could connect with your adversary in combat is a fulcrum for force. Practice such that you make use of these fulcrums to uplift and move the whole of your body.[107]

Master Ren, I would like to ask, how does one go about "using the mind to control the body?" Can you please explain the specific requirements that must be met in order to do this? Should each and every move in a *taijiquan* form be executed by "using the mind to control the body?"

First you must attain unity of all parts of your body. In the early stages, use your mind to conduct the actions of your waist. Your waist will drive your *shen* and *qi*, and your *shen* and *qi* will drive your whole body. Gradually you will come to sense that the entirety of your body is directed and powered in unison from its centerline. Later on, your mind need only stir in order for your whole body to respond. That is the way it should be, including within any small movement you execute.

*Qi* is something that can only be sensed and known—there is no way to describe it. Here, although I follow along with the modern custom of using the character *qi* instead of *Qi*, I do not merely refer to the *qi* of the body that *qigong* emphasizes. *Taijiquan* requires everything inside and outside of the body to be transformed into *shen* and *qi*. If you become attached to the interior of the body, how will your whole body become open and connected?

---

[107] This statement seems to contradict earlier statements that the waist should always act as the fulcrum. Ren clarified this point for me, saying "this means that once one can already use the waist to control the body it is no longer necessary to pay attention to the waist."

Master Ren, please elucidate the following passage: "The whole body needs to be equipollent and expansive; there can be no places where strength is contracted. Gathered strength is expansive strength; it is not contracted strength.[108] If there is any contracted strength, then everything is worthless. The hardest place to achieve equipollence and expansion is the knees. Once the knees are equipollent and expansive, everywhere else will be, too. If the knees are braced, the shoulders will not open, and nor will the space within the chest and abdomen." Does contracted strength refer to force gathered in the body, or something else?

Gathering is the concentration of force. *Shen, qi,* and force can concentrate, but the physical body must be equipollent and expansive like a great surging wave or soaring bluffs.

In *taijiquan* you definitely do not first draw in the body in order to spring open. The type of strength used by a master of *taijiquan* has its basis in the concentration and release of *shen* and *qi*. The importance of this point cannot be overstated. You must not misunderstand it. I recommend you try examining Master Yang Chengfu's bearing in old photographs of him touching hands with other people to get a *feel* for what I am trying to describe.

You've asked a very good question—that you have grasped this much indicates that you already have one foot on the path. It leaves me with no small amount of remorse that I am not better able to express these things in writing.

---

[108] Master Ren explained that "contracted strength" here refers to the tendency of people who are using musculoskeletal strength to crouch and contract their bodies in order to prepare to try and explode outward.

CHAPTER 5   123

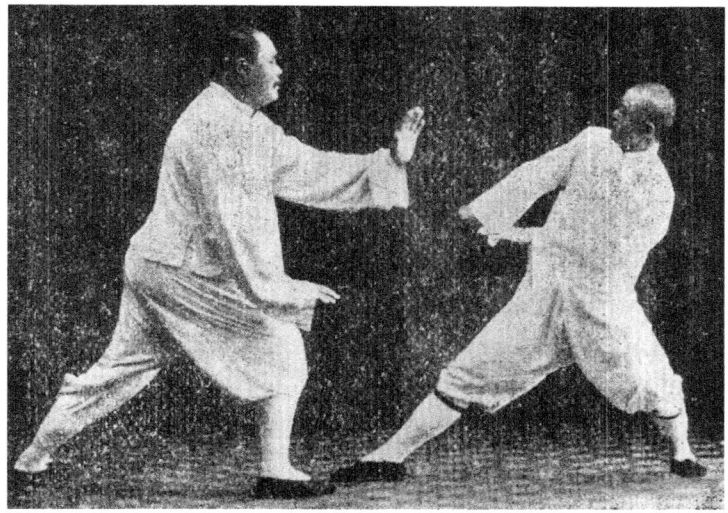

Yang Chengfu demonstrating sparring

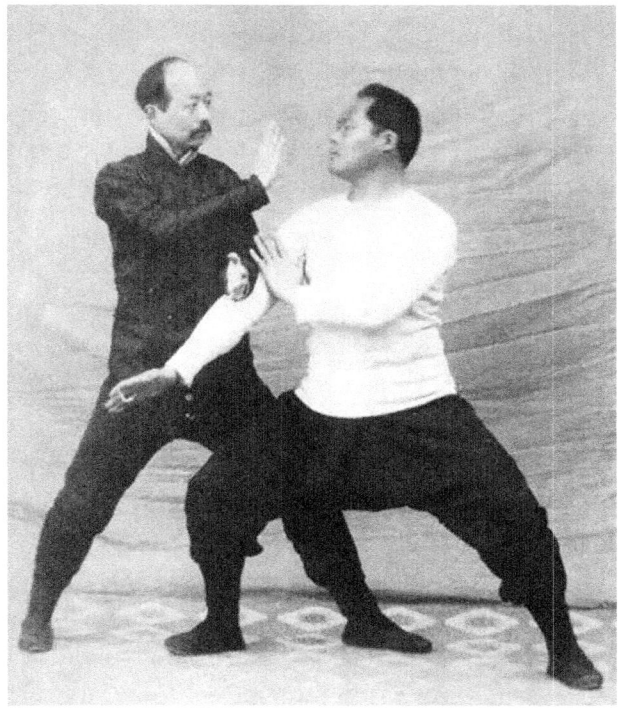

Yang Chengfu demonstrating sparring in his youth

You said, "The first thing to do is train in order to link all parts of your body into an equipollent unity that responds in its entirety the very instant your waist moves. You'll only be able to work with your body's weight once you have reached this stage. When your waist can act like a sort of director general that powers the rest of the body, you're ready." I'm afraid that these sentences are a bit lacking in practicability. *Taijiquan* is indeed a form of whole-body movement, but you do not necessarily need to stress that the waist fulfills an absolute function in the movement of the entire physique. Your emphasis is perhaps due to your own specific way of doing things. According to my own experience, if one were to emphasize a specific area's importance, one would say that *taijiquan*'s flexibility derives from the pelvis. Strength, however, does not come solely from the waist. What one should actually feel is that the entire body is open and connected. If there is a point of attachment—for instance, if one feels that one's power is in one's waist—then I'm afraid that one is not living up to the ethos of "using intent, not using strength." Some might ask, is it acceptable to have the waist be the place where one "uses intent?" Well, my experience leads me to conclude that the best approach is to remain unattached to any specific bodily region. I do not know whether I am correct or not, so please favor me with your advice.

The waist's role is something that beginners cannot ignore. Of course, if you have developed consummate skill, then you need not place your attention upon the lumbar region.

In *taijiquan* training, one must learn to unite the power that commands the body, because in the very beginning students are incapable of having their bodies and minds function in unison. If one's hope is that the body will listen to the mind's commands, then it is necessary to start by learning how to have the whole body's *shen* and *qi* follow the waist's lead. This is akin to summoning the disbanded, wandering conscripts of the body to train together in boot camp, and it is the only way to gradually become capable of having *shen, qi,* and the body respond the instant the mind moves. This training process is indispensable.

In answer to your comment that flexibility derives from the pelvis, I must reiterate that agility comes when a practitioner of *taijiquan* goes from moving primarily via the musculoskeletal system to moving primarily via *shen* and *qi*. This is what is implied by the phrase "emptily guiding strength upwards." A supple pelvis will only increase the body's relative agility. It should not be viewed as an intrinsic aspect of *taijiquan* and the internal martial arts. Other martial arts actually have superior methods for training this part of the body.

Previously, with regard to what happens after a practitioner has opened his or her skeletature and united the body, you said "at that point if you counter an external force you'll have a root beneath your feet and the fulcrum where you receive this stress will be in your waist instead of in your shoulders or your chest. You will then be able to withstand very strong force within a state of relaxation." I beg to differ with your opinion that "the fulcrum where you receive the stress of an external force will be in your waist." When there is an external force, all joints in the body should act as fulcrums that roundly take the stress upon themselves.

This issue is one that many people have trouble wrapping their minds around, and it also frequently comes up as a point of contention in debates about skill levels. The confusion largely arises because nowadays people only compare skill by pushing hands, whereas our predecessors engaged in actual combat when they compared their skill with wandering martial artists and the like. What you generally see in push hands these days is that as soon as the person of lesser skill receives external force, it will get lodged in his or her back, shoulders, or chest. When this happens, the practitioner can do little more than passively receive a beating. When the participant of greater skill receives external force, it naturally moves into his or her heels or even a meter beneath his or her feet. Those with advanced skill are able to absorb a push coming from numerous people at the same time without falling over, but this only works when everybody is so committed to the push that they refrain from using their hands to strike and their feet to kick. When demonstrating such a skill the practitioner dares not compromise his or her posture by even an inch, so we have to wonder, is there any use for such a technique in actual fighting? This is why we don't see any record of the three original Yang family masters and their highly achieved students demonstrating skills like this. Suppose that while doing so a third party wielding a blade made an attack—what could you do?

Regarding the discussion of being rooted under the feet when receiving an external force, my experience is that there is utterly no need to receive force—just as ever, I make it empty and then I return it to my opponent. However much I take, I return. Why would I receive it? All is resolved in the amount of time it takes for lightning to strike or two pieces of flint to create a spark.

When one is *song* one can bear extremely powerful external force. One can relaxedly sink an opponent's strength beneath one's own feet, even guiding it down to great depths. But that will never be superior to making it empty and returning it to the opponent. If one has the habit of emptying and returning force, should a third party attack with a knife when one is already engaged in combat, one will be free to calmly turn and deal with the new threat.

Push hands has always been a training method in *taijiquan*, and nowadays it has turned into a means of exchange between practitioners, but it can never stand in for real contact sparring. A person who is genuinely capable of *not* receiving external force has already entered the door and possesses real internal martial arts skill, but this comes after passing through the early stages of practice. The early stages are still important, so those of us who have passed beyond them should not destroy the ladder, as it were. Rather, it is our responsibility to make sure the ladder remains standing in good repair for future students to climb.

Master Ren, my understanding is that in *taijiquan* practice it is easy to get "stuck" with fulcrums formed in incorrect places such as the chest, shoulders, knees, abdomen, and so forth. When this happens, it becomes impossible to make progress in one's training, so one must therefore get "stuck" on the lumbar vertebrae region. Is this correct?

In *taijiquan*'s training of the waist, one begins by learning to subtly uplift the *mingmen* point on the waist (not the entirety of the lumbar vertebrae). Eventually anywhere the mind is placed will be able to drive the whole body, and the feeling of an internal centerline will take shape. When these changes occur, they do not occur at the level of the flesh and bones.

"Equipollent and expansive" do not refer merely to relaxing and extending. These words imply training so that the entire body becomes *song*, such that the physical body's movements manifest equipollently. This is different from musculoskeletal movements that are powered by flexing the muscles. Strength is something that all people have, but the strength of those who train internal martial arts is amplified by way of unity. The average person's strength is diminished by discord and disunity.

Master Ren, I have two more questions I would like to ask you today. The first is regarding the task of "learning to subtly uplift the *mingmen* point on the waist." May I interpret this as meaning that after I slightly poke my buttocks forward, the center of the roughly circular region of my waist will naturally stick out a bit further than it would under normal circumstances? Secondly, you stated that the "physical body's movements manifest equipollently." This notion is very difficult to understand, whereas the idea of "musculoskeletal movements that are powered by flexing the muscles" is much easier to grasp. Is there a simpler way you could put "equipollence" into words for us?

Firstly, "straightening the waist" is exactly the opposite of what you describe. What you describe is sticking out the waist. In Yang style *taijiquan* there has only ever been the instruction to straighten the waist. I am not sure where the later idea of poking out the *mingmen* region came from.

Secondly, if you melt away the stiff places in your body, then you will feel as though your body possesses evenly distributed uniformity (like a liquid or a gas). Once you have this experience, then it becomes quite easy to understand what is meant by "equipollence."

When you say, "If you melt away the stiff places in your body, then you will feel as though your body possesses evenly distributed uniformity (like a liquid or a gas)," what shape does this "evenly distributed uniformity" take on? Is it globular?

As your *shen* and *qi* slowly become replete, your body will gradually start to feel as though it were part and parcel with *shen* and *qi*. When engaged in combat, a body with uniformity can transform as per the heart's desire. It need not be rounded, nor need it be angular.

Master Ren, earlier you were asked about the phrase, "The whole body needs to be equipollent and expansive; there can be no places where strength is contracted... The hardest place to achieve equipollence and expansion is the knees." How exactly is equipollence achieved?

Regardless of whether you are gathering or expelling power, you should not be simply contracting and releasing your muscles. Rather, your body should be as one, and in both stillness and movement your *shen* and *qi* should always be equipollent.

Master Ren, is "equipollence" something that occurs at the level of thought and consciousness?

Start by training bodily equipollence, and then slowly start to use equipollence of *shen* and *qi* to gradually turn your body into an aspect of *shen* and *qi* that moves equipollently in concert with the mind. This is not a question of thought.

Earlier you wrote, "There is utterly no need to receive force—just as ever, I make it empty and then I return it to my opponent. However much I take, I return. Why would I receive it?" How is this done? Does it mean treating external force as intent and *qi* and then sending it back into an opponent in an arc?

When you are able to feel as though your body is levitating and no longer connected to the earth, and moreover that the movements of your *shen*, *qi*, and body are becoming freer and freer, then naturally you will cease to get stuck by opponents' strength. If you have not yet arrived at that level do not try to contrive this ability, or else you may end up with imaginary *taijiquan*. Given that *taijiquan* is a martial art, it needs to be functional in real life combat. Trying to use your mind to grasp these things is dangerous, so instead you should seek to train diligently in accord with the principles of this art. If you do, when the time is ripe, your skill will reach maturity.

The words of past masters can be used to verify our experiences, but beware of drawing false conclusions on the basis of them. Learning to have the waist act as a fulcrum is a process that takes time. In the end, it leads towards placing the fulcrum in the heels. Only when you are able to make your entire body open, interconnected, and free of any points at which strength becomes stuck are you truly doing things correctly. Before that point, *always* have your waist be in command, and then gradually the stiff places in your body will leave your body through your feet. Conversely, if you focus your attention upon your heels, you will never shed the stiffness in your body.

Master Ren, you said, "One slowly comes to feel that where the mind is placed lies a centerline that is empty, numinous, and capable of changing in ways that conduct the motions of the whole body. Later still, one will feel that this centerline can change positions and that it comprises the mind and not the muscles or the skeleton. This is what Master Sun Lutang was referring to when he said 'anywhere in my body can act as the fulcrum, and thus there is no limit to the ways in which I can transform.'" Does this centerline comprised of the mind refer to a line in the body that is perpendicular to the ground and centered upon the waist?

Given that this centerline's arrival is predicated by the concentration of the mind, the question of whether it is centered upon the waist or not is irrelevant. Its location can be changed at will, and thus in the movement "a needle on the seafloor" it is in the hands.[109] Nevertheless, everything I just described begins with working on the waist. When conditions are allowed to ripen, advancements come effortlessly.

Master Ren, you wrote, "Very subtly straighten up the *mingmen* area on the waist. Make use of this upward-lifting strength so that the whole body is *song* and open." Won't doing this cause the waist to become tense and stiff?

The key idea here is to *subtly* straighten the waist. In the beginning this requires some effort, but eventually your waist will stay straight even without you devoting attention to the task. Nevertheless, you still need to carefully maintain a sense of empty agility in the waist and try your best not to let the area become stiff.

    There can be endless discussion of the finer details, but in the end the point of all of this is nurturing *qi*. The elimination of stiffness

---

[109] Movements with this name exist in many *taijiquan* forms, including Yang style forms. In Chinese it is written "海底针."

in the body begins with *zhanzhuang*. The lengthening of soft tissues and expanding of the skeletature starts with the pelvis. Not having a teacher to demonstrate this power in person will slow your progress. The best thing you can do is work on your foundation until the opportunity arises for you to study with a qualified *taijiquan* teacher.

How are the mind and the physical body merged? Once they are merged, if one attacks an adversary, does the mind arrive before the physical body does? Is there a time delay? Thank you.

One must be able to distinguish body and mind in order to merge them. The more *song* the body is, the more quickly body and mind will unite. At later stages, it is as though the body is a component of *shen* and *qi*, and the two effectively move at the same speed.

Master Ren, would you please teach me how to "nurture *qi*?" Does this imply standing in the *wuji zhanzhuang* posture or other forms of training where the body is not moving, such as seated meditation or practicing the small and large heavenly circulations?

There are two types of *qi*, which the ancients wrote as *qi* and *Qi*. One's foundation comes from the post-heavenly "*qi*" derived from food. The foremost way to nurture *qi* is to practice a lot while maintaining a balanced lifestyle. The keys to nurturing *qi* lie in going to sleep by 11pm or so, sleeping for eight hours, and maintaining a clear mind with few desires.

When post-heavenly *qi* is replete, it gathers in the *dantian* as *jing* and *qi*. One must be enlightened to the principle of *wuji* in order to transform *jing* and *qi* into prior heavenly "*Qi*." Nourishing prior heaven *Qi* in the *wuji* state while doing martial arts training, *zhanzhuang*, and practices performed in stillness is the only way to step over the threshold into the realm of internal martial arts.

My interpretation and what I have experienced in practice is that one exhales and expels while "straightening" the waist, whereas when "drawing in" the waist one inhales and gathers. Master Ren, is my understanding correct?

Your waist needs to be subtly lifted during both gathering and expelling, so you should always have the sense that your waist is straight. However, be aware that this is an empty, sprightly sort of straightening. You should never feel like you are straightening it unto a point of rigidity.

For the last few months I have had the feeling that my body is like a uniform liquid, and yet my joints are far from being as open as they should be. Please tell me what I should emphasize at this stage while I am training. What kind of problems should I pay attention to? Thank you!

Congratulations—you've arrived at a pretty good place. Right now you should at all times pay attention to your lumbar region while training. Do not place your attention on your joints. As you have built a foundation, they will melt open soon enough.

Does one need to brace oneself with strength in order to effect the "melting" open of the joints? Or should one simply maintain "a state like a uniform liquid," refrain from bracing, constantly pay attention to the waist, and thereby gradually "melt?"

You cannot brace yourself with strength. Any and all contrived efforts cause the body to harden.

Master Ren, please would you tell me whether or not in Yang style *taijiquan* one should "move the groin along an arc?" Also, I have heard it said that "one should move like a boat carrying a heavy load." What do you make of that analogy?

The first idea comes from Chen style *taijiquan*, which I have not studied, so I am not entirely sure what it means to have the groin move along an arc. I do think the second analogy is quite apt, though.

Master Ren, can you explain in detail how to "constantly pay attention to the waist?" Also, when "treating the waist as an axis," is there a difference between vertical and horizontal axes?

The waist is always the force that governs and controls the body. Treating it as an axis is a mistake, as axis and controller are two entirely different things.

Sometimes when I am uplifting my waist I will cause my *qi* to rise or I will suck in my belly in spite of the fact that I have no intention of doing so. Please explain how I might resolve this problem.

When you uplift the waist, it should be as though a hand clasped around your lumbar spine is leading the movements of your entire body. Thus, as you lift the waist, your abdomen, back, and every other part of your body are all *song*.
    Before your waist is capable of acting as the force that commands your entire body, do not prematurely try to uplift the waist.

I've been studying *taijiquan* for less than a month using Master Cui Zhongsan's 108-move traditional Yang style form video lessons. I seem to have vaguely gotten the knack for "sinking the shoulders and letting the elbows drop," but after I've trained awhile the areas between my shoulders and my neck become very stiff.

You might be making a mistake when you practice. "*Song*" refers to relaxing and opening. When done correctly, your interior will possess flow, and the space beneath your armpits will be open as though you were clutching two hot steamed buns under your arms. You must not let your relaxation turn into flaccidity. In a flaccid or floppy state your interior is not connected—rather, it is simply deflated. This is an area where many people go astray. Be careful to avoid training incorrectly.

While following the instruction to "straighten the waist," as one empties one leg and shifts bodyweight into the other, should the *mingmen* point on the waist be split into two separate points?

There is only ever one *mingmen*. When first learning to straighten your waist you start with a single point. Later, this point will grow to include the whole segment of your waist beneath your *mingmen*, and this area will act as the controller of your whole body. When this occurs, that will mean you have accomplished the first step in cultivating the waist.

What books on *taijiquan* do you recommend to beginners?

Read Master Li Yaxuan's book![110] As for photos, study the ones taken of Master Yang Chengfu.

---

[110] Li Yaxuan's book is entitled 《太極拳學論》 (*Tai Ji Quan Xue Lun* or *Treatises On the Study of Taijiquan*). It has not yet been translated into English.

While I am training *taijiquan* stances it feels especially difficult to relax my chest and upper back. The whole region feels like a single plank of wood. Master Ren, can you please tell me how I can get my thoracic vertebrae as well as the rest of my spine to be *song* and open?

Fusion in the thoracic region is very difficult to melt open, so a long period of committed training is unavoidable. Spend more time allowing yourself to directly experience the principle that your body is thoroughly penetrated by emptiness.[111]

Is it okay to cross train *taijiquan* and dumbbell workouts? Is it advisable to add weight to the body while training *zhanzhuang*?

Do not hold extra weight while practicing *zhanzhuang*, or else you will cultivate the sort of strength one gets from holding the breath and exerting oneself. For the same reason, avoid cross training *taijiquan* and dumbbell routines.

Master Ren, what type of posture should beginning students of *zhanzhuang* practice with? Should we choose *wuji* posture *zhanzhuang*, or *taiji* posture *zhanzhuang*? Or would a hand-brushes-knee stance be better?[112] Should our waists be straightened forwards, or should our lumbar regions push out backwards? How do we maintain an upright and symmetrical posture while "straightening the waist?"

---

[111] Master Ren added the following elaboration of this instruction when we discussed this portion of the text in person: "At all times, even when one is exerting strength or having strength be exerted upon oneself, one should always feel as though one's body is empty."

[112] "搂膝拗步," the name of a posture found in many *taijiquan* forms.

Straightening the waist is done to establish the body's center of command—its only goal is to ensure that the waist is capable of controlling the whole body. If the waist is straightened unto a point of stiffness, other parts of the body will not be able to relax, so excessive straightening is mistaken. If you keep it firmly in mind that straightening the waist is done in order to facilitate a state of *song* and openness throughout the whole of your body, as well as to create a fulcrum and center of command for your body, then any sort of *zhanzhuang* posture is just fine!

When straightening the waist, the *mingmen* area is pulled upwards and towards the front of your body. There is no basis to the assertion that the *mingmen* area should be pushed outwards.

The deciding factor when it comes to whether or not your *taijiquan* practice will allow you to "enter the door" lies in the waist. The process of developing the waist is more or less as follows: first you straighten out the *mingmen* area so that it becomes the controller and governor of your entire body, capable of supporting your own body weight in addition to external forces coming from opponents. In time, just below the *mingmen* (at a distance of one finger width or so) a small region that obviously commands and governs the body will slowly make its presence known. After it has appeared, you then train in using it to lift and make *song* your entire body.

If you attempt to lift your whole body via the *mingmen* as I just described from the very beginning, it is very likely that you will mistakenly angle your waist upwards and backwards, thereby slamming shut the door to the internal martial arts. There is no shortage of people out there who train *taijiquan* incorrectly. A big part of the reason they are looked down upon by practitioners of other martial arts is that they lack unimpeded, integral power. Much in the way that a lion cub is given a wide berth by other animals in spite of being far from realizing its potential strength and grandeur, a person who has truly "entered the door" will not be looked down on, even if he or she has a long way to go before mastery.

Your doubts and confusion will vanish the day you enter the door. If, after five or six years of training, you are still plagued by doubt, then there is no question that the path you have taken is mistaken. Five or six years of dedication to external martial arts, grappling arts, or boxing will produce a level of proficiency. Even more should this be the case with *taijiquan*, which is one of the crown jewels of the internal martial arts!

In sum, as soon as you catch a glimpse of the real, you will be left with no more room for uncertainty. If uncertainty continues to haunt you, this simply means you have yet to encounter authentic *taijiquan*.

---

Of late I have suffered from headaches where my head feels swollen and under pressure and my memory suffers. Neither western medicine nor traditional Chinese medicine has offered much help, so now I'm giving *taijiquan* a try with an open mind. However, when I practice *zhanzhuang* I find that my mind never relaxes, so I am hopeful that you can offer me a few recommendations.

---

Your symptoms suggest a mind that is scattered and chaotic, which might have been brought on by overthinking the problems in your life. When you practice, do not contemplate any theoretical principles, and do not pay attention to the sensations that arise or the states that you may experience. Twice each day, practice standing in a low horse stance, once in the morning and once in the evening. While keeping your torso perpendicular to the ground, attempt to maintain as low of a posture as you can, with your waist subtly straightened upwards. Do your best to relax the rest of your body and keep the angle of your groin wide open and your pelvis rounded. Each time, stand like this until the pain in your legs is so great that it's impossible to continue, and then stand up. During each of your morning and evening sessions repeat this process a total of three times. After a week your condition should improve. You can also light agarwood incense while you train to help calm your spirits.

I'm afraid the cause of my headaches is probably not as simple as you suggest; after all, I have suffered from them for more than a year. Nevertheless, I will give training according to your suggestions a go. I have been practicing the *wuji zhanzhuang* stance. Does this mean I should leave the stance more or less the same, aside from attempting to bend my legs as much as possible? Should my legs be further apart? Are there any specific things I should do when initiating or closing the practice?

For now, you should not use the *wuji* posture, because until you have developed *gongfu* in the lower region of your body, whatever *qi* you cultivate will simply add energy to your scattered, chaotic thinking. Lacking *gongfu* in the lower portion of the body is a major reason people who only practice stillness and do not practice movement methods frequently develop problems. Putting the lower half of your body under some strain should quickly ameliorate your symptoms.

There is an old saying, "Those who understand principles have nothing to fear; those who can restrain themselves have nothing to worry about."[113] I would like to know, how does one achieve the second half of this saying?

"Those who can restrain themselves have nothing to worry about" is an idea with roots in Confucian character cultivation. It means that if you eliminate inappropriate habits of thinking, then you will become magnanimous and free from anxiety.

---

[113] From "明理則不懼，尅己則無憂."

Can you please explain in detail what you mean when you say "your *shen* and *qi* will surge into empty spaces like lightning?"

Once *shen* and *Qi* are fully refined, your mind will concentrate with blade-like acuity. When in a state of expansion, *shen* and *qi* cut inwards.[114]

Master Ren, please tell me what the fundamental considerations of *taijiquan* practice are.

An outline of the basic requirements and processes found in *taijiquan* is as follows:

(1) Firstly, straighten the waist, open the angle of the groin, and round out the pelvis through *zhanzhuang* and other foundational exercises. Use these practices to lift and *song* the whole body, melt away its areas of stiffness, give the body a unified point of control, and to integrate the upper and lower halves of your musculoskeletal system. Provided that you learn authentic methods and use them properly, if you train in this manner for two to three years, then success is inevitable! Success at this stage means that when you encounter an external force, there is a root beneath your feet, and the fulcrum receiving the force is in your waist instead of in your shoulders, chest, or anywhere else. At this point, when in a state of *song*, you will be able to withstand an extraordinary amount of external force.

(2) Subsequently you must train *shen* and *qi*, using your mind to move *qi*, and using *qi* to move your body. Gradually your hands and feet, the rest of your body, and your *shen* and *qi* will all follow your mind in unison. This is described as "*shen* and *qi* are the sovereign; bones and flesh are the loyal ministers." To reach this stage requires

---

[114] Ren used both 炁 and 氣 in his answer. I have preserved his wording.

approximately another two years. Once you are here, you are truly practicing internal martial arts. If you use the principles of mutual restraint and generation from the five phases to move your body, your *shen*, and your *qi*, then what you are doing is *wuxingquan*; if you use the eight trigram principle of transformation to move your body, your *shen*, and your *qi*, then what you are doing is called *baguazhang*. If you wish to learn *taiji*, then you must first understand the principle of *wuji* and directly experience the concept of being of one body with all things. This point is very difficult—it requires you firstly to have a basis in traditional Chinese cultural knowledge, secondly to have ample *shen* and *qi*, and finally to have a qualified teacher point you in the correct direction. These criteria must be met for it to be possible for you to have hope of directly experiencing the subtle.

If luck shines upon you and you have an epiphany, then you must carefully maintain this state in order to give it time to mature. If you arrive at this stage, then regardless of how strong or enormous your opponent might be, you will not give rise to thoughts of reacting. Rather, you and your adversary will be of one and the same *wuji*, within which you can freely move in offense or defense without damaging the *wuji* principle. It is when you have reached this level that your foundation in *taijiquan* can finally be used.

Later still, you must perceive how your opponent's movements within this *wuji* create an energetic change that seeks to destroy the *wuji*. This energetic disturbance is described as "insubstantiality and substantiality." It is none other than *taiji*, which is born of *wuji* when movement creates the divergence of *yin* and *yang*.

Subsequently, pick apart the theories in Wang Zongyue's *Treatise on Taijiquan* and watch as your world is born anew. It is extremely difficult to awaken to the *wuji* principle. Some devote their lives to this pursuit and yet fail to enter the door. Failure and success have a relationship with one's foundation in Confucian, Buddhist, and Daoist philosophy.

(3) The above information pertains to the different requirements and practices for *taijiquan* training at each stage. Because each stu-

dent's physical condition and imbalances are different, in practice the specifics of what is listed above have to be modified in accord with individuals' constitutions. However, modifications are only made in pursuit of the goalposts I just detailed.

I still cannot figure out what "opening" and "closing" are. Do these words refer to the mind and *shen*'s opening and closing, or that of intent and *qi*? Or do opening and closing have something to do with the movements of the physical body? For example, you wrote, "When gathering inhale. As you inhale, mind and *shen* merge, while intent and *qi* expand." You also wrote, "*Shen* and *qi* cut inwards while in a state of openness." Do these sentences describe instances where the practitioner himself or herself is in an equipollent state?

When I wrote about mind and *shen*, intent and *qi*, and power, I was referring to the practitioner's own state. For now I recommend only that you avoid thinking too much about questions that pertain to fairly late stages in training. First cultivate your own *shen* and *qi*. In time you will naturally come to know and understand the nature of these issues.

You said in order to "give the body a unified point of control, and to integrate the upper and lower halves of your musculoskeletal system," one must first relax and open four major joints: the two shoulders and the two hips. My understanding is that once the hip joints are *song*, it is as though the *dantian* is atop a platform, and therefore the opposing pulling forces coming from the two hips will power the *dantian*'s internal rotation, which is then conducted out to the distal joints. Is this correct?

Actually, in *taijiquan* training, so long as you straighten your waist, open up your pelvis, round out your groin, and use your centerline to uplift and *song* your whole body, then your shoulders and hips will gradually relax and open of their own accord. Moreover, one day you will suddenly feel that your hands are connected to your centerline, after which point any external force your arms encounter will cease to get stuck in your shoulders or chest. Instead, your hands will naturally move your opponent or transform the external force. Then one day your legs will also suddenly connect to your centerline, and then all four of your limbs will feel like an octopus' tentacles.[115] At that point it is said that a practitioner does not even need to know how his or her arms and legs are moving.

If you try to intentionally relax your shoulders and hips then you will not arrive at the level I just described. The reason is that if your individual limbs are under intentional control, then they will never submit to the center of control in the waist.

When the weather is good, how many times should I train my *taijiquan* form? How should I nurture *qi*? How can I become so tranquil that nothing around me is not tranquil? Other than thinking about things to illuminate their principles, what other common methods are there?

Regardless of whether the weather is clement or not, do not let there be breaks in your training. If you are busy you can practice less, but you should not skip practice altogether. Water will only reach the boil if the fire beneath it burns steadily; if the stove is sometimes hot and sometimes cold, the water will never boil.

The best way to nurture *qi* is to clarify your mind and diminish your desires.

Awakenings to the principles of *taijiquan* occur very suddenly, but these sudden awakenings reciprocate with the gradual process of your training. As your skills slowly improve, because your body will

---

[115] In conversation Master Ren mentioned that this an imperfect analogy, so readers should not take it too literally.

respond to the principles at work, your insights will both deepen as well as become more concrete.

I have been training my *shen*, intent, and *qi* for a year. My physical stances meet the basic requirements, but I still tend to lack confidence and worry that I am practicing a fake martial art. Please tell me how I can prove to myself that these things are real.

Encountering authentic *taijiquan* will leave you with absolutely no room for doubt. That you currently lack confidence indicates you definitely have a problem. The best way to resolve your problem and prove things to yourself is to be able to perform entirely in accord with the treatises on *taijiquan* written by the old masters. If you can do so, you will be indomitable.

I believe in the formidability of *shen*, intent, and *qi*, because I have seen them in action. When I am training *taijiquan* on my own I feel that these things are real, but when I attempt to apply them with an opponent I am not particularly formidable. Please tell me, is there a difference between training the forms and directly using *shen*, intent, and *qi*?

Training *taijiquan* forms is like grinding a blade upon a whetstone. Combat is putting the blade to use, but this can only be done once both your *shen* and your body follow the very instant your mind moves. If you have to stand and think before you move your mind, and when you finally move your mind your body can't keep up, then you are not ready for combat. The old saying that "one must train *taiji* for a decade before leaving the gate" probably addresses this issue. When your skills have truly arrived you will no longer be in doubt. Right now, you're as unconfident as you would be if you were trying to cross a murky river by feeling for stepping stones with your toes.

Visualizing an opponent standing before you is a must when practicing *taijiquan*. Form training and actual fighting are one and the same thing. If they were not one and the same, how could you hope for your *shen* and your body to follow your mind when the time came for you to actually use *taijiquan* in self-defense?

I am a new student of Zhao Bao *taijiquan*.[116] As I am not an "inner door" student, I am not entirely clear about *taijiquan*'s training methods and the sequence of their practice. Master Ren, please tell me what steps I should take in my training right now. Thank you!

In the beginning, you should start with some foundation-building exercises, and from there you need to start to treat your waist as the central commanding force in your body, in addition to making your whole body *song* and open. In principle, you should have some foundation before you begin training a *taijiquan* form. The purpose of doing forms is to maintain and deepen your *gongfu* while you are in a state of motion.

Master Ren, an essay on *taijiquan* states, "In order to train the spine, one must first practice *quan*,[117] *qing*,[118] *yin*,[119] *song*, and *fang*,[120] to link up each vertebra one by one." Can you please explain the implications of this sentence and the relevant training methods? Are these things meant to be performed in sequence, or are they all obtained simply by constantly using the waist as the governor of the body?

---

[116] A school of *taijiquan* named after the martial artist Zhao Bao.

[117] "拳" literally means "fist" and is often used to mean "martial art," but Master Ren said that in this context it refers to the "process" of training.

[118] "擎" literally means "to lift up," but here it is a reference to getting an opponent to "step into emptiness," at which point it is *as though* one is lifting him or her up.

[119] "引," "to guide," here means to use force (勢) to move one's opponent.

[120] "放," "to release," here means to expel stored force.

As you train in having your waist be your body's center of control, your vertebra will naturally come to feel fully linked up. Once they do, then you can go on and specifically train *qing*, *yin*, *song*, and *fang*.

Master Ren, can you please tell me whether or not you specifically train in the "outer three unities?"[121] At what stage is it a good idea to train the outer three unities?

In my training I only pay attention to the unity of the body with *shen* and *qi*. I do not pay attention to anything else.

Having read over several of your writings, I've discovered that you repeatedly emphasize the importance of opening the groin, rounding out the pelvis, and straightening the waist when addressing beginners. Can you speak about the angle of the buttocks, whether or not to lift the anal sphincter, and the angle of the waist when it is being straightened?

Do not angle your buttocks forward or pull up your anal sphincter. When straightened, your waist should be angled slightly forwards, never backwards. Please take a look at the photos of Master Yang Chengfu training when he was young, as his stances convey more wisdom than my words can.

---

[121] This term, "外三合," usually refers to connectedness of the elbows, knees, and hip joints.

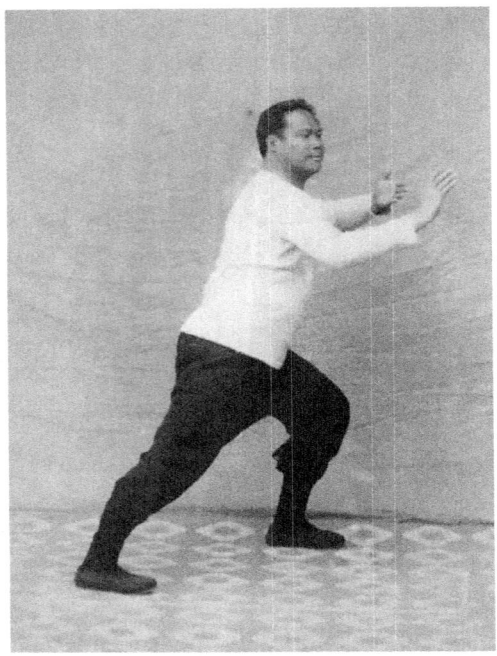

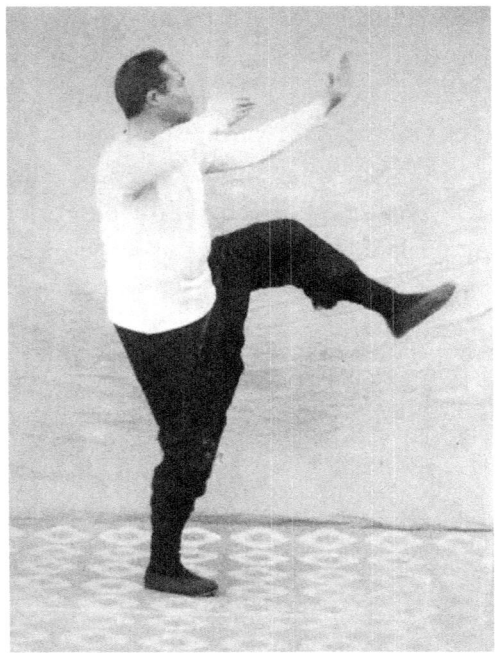

Yang Chengfu

Master Ren, you state that attention should be placed upon a point on the waist during *taijiquan* practice, but the *Treatise on Taijiquan* also requires students to "stand like a balance scale." The latter requirement indicates that suspending the top of the head is also very important. Should we pay attention to suspending the top of the head when we're training? Also, can you please describe the types of power present in *peng, an, lü,* and *ji*?

Before you are adept at training your waist you cannot suspend the top of your head, you can only fake it. Suspending the top of your head will only be real *after* you have completed training your waist. At this point, your head's suspension will grow from your waist.[122]

Regarding your second question: *Peng*'s power is like the emptiness within a flame. *An*'s power is like the fullness of a river running in a downward torrent. *Lü*'s power is like molten metal on the brink of dripping downwards. *Ji*'s power is like an ancient tree when it first began growing. You have my apologies—it's truly impossible to concretely describe these things in words!

---

[122] Ren said to me that it will feel as though there is a central line that controls the entire body arising from the waist. He emphasized that this is a sensation, not a thing. Moreover, this sensation will make it seem as though there is a line that holds the head and all beneath it relaxed and at one with the space around oneself. The feeling is one of having a center. Anticipating readers' potential questions, I asked Master Ren if this sensation has any relationship with the central channel cultivated in some yogic disciplines. He said he does not know.

What is your opinion of this photo taken of Yang Chengfu training when he was in his youth?

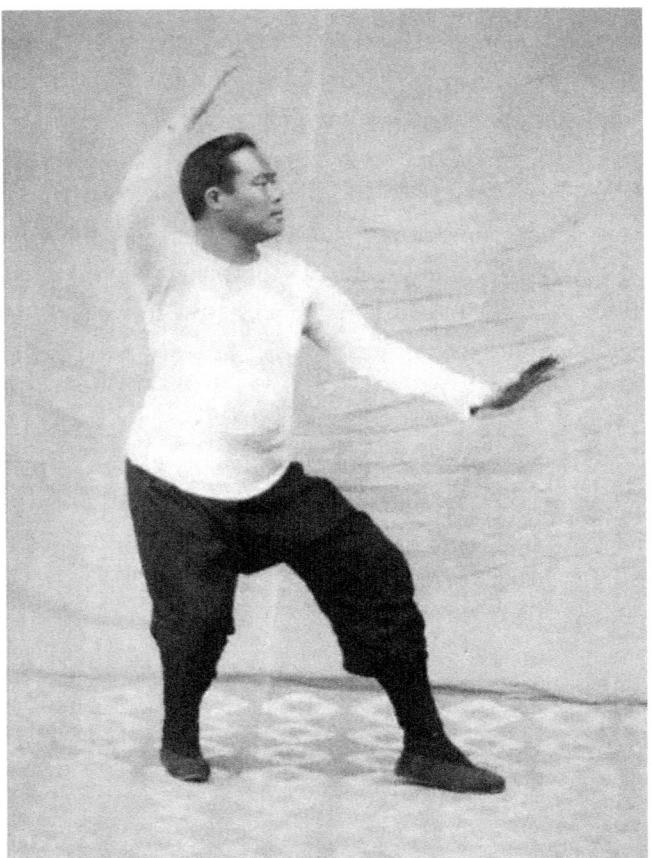

Yang Chengfu

This photo is a real treasure. It was taken before Master Yang's *gongfu* was fully accomplished, but from it we can glimpse hints of how he trained. Specifically, it shows us the way for beginners to straighten their waists. It is much harder to find similar hints in photos taken of Master Yang later in life, when he was truly an adept, so the most we can do is admire them.

Master Ren, after reading the eight essays on *taijiquan* written by Master Yue Huanzhi's son, Yue Tan,[123] my takeaway can be summed up with a single word: wholeness. There is one passage in his essays that very succinctly reflects this word: "One's body is as though round and borderless, yet within one's body there is contained an angularity that is impossible to pin down. Within transformation is contained melting; within yielding there is standing firm. One's *qi* emerges from the mind, one's strength emerges from intent. Please, carefully begin with the waist, as though you were newly pregnant. Beginners must not fail to value this instruction. You must seek to train your physique in accord with the principles. When the time is ripe, your skills will mature. You must not force things, either internally or externally. Holistically move your intent, never disconnecting from your skeletature and musculature. Those on the highest plane are as though egoless. *Taiji* is *wuji*." I began my training according to my understanding of Yue Tan's instructions, but I am not sure whether or not my understanding is on point, so please tell me what you think. Also, I have begun training on the basis of Master Li Deyin's books. Are there any potential problems I might need to be wary of? I bow in thanks.

Your interpretation is spot on. As for whether or not you're really managing to train in accord with these principles, I have no way of saying. Nevertheless, that you have benefited from Yue Tan's essays is a good thing. With respect to Master Li Deyin (who was a disciple of Yang Shouzhong), although I have met him I have never seen his *taijiquan* in action, so I can make no qualified statements about him or his books. In any event, it is always best to be taught directly by a qualified teacher. I find it difficult to believe anybody could master the martial arts solely on the basis of reading books.

---

[123] Yue Tan, who was Yue Huanzhi's son, wrote 《太極拳要義》 (*Tai Ji Quan Yao Yi*, or *The Essential Meaning of Taijiquan*), a tract containing eight essays on *taijiquan*.

I have been practicing *taijiquan* for five years, but only very recently have I begun to truly sense *taiji*'s internal *qi* and pathways of strength.[124] On account of these new sensations I have a rather bold question I would like to ask you. Specifically, given that I am a person of the world who partakes of worldly activities, how should I address my sexual appetites if I wish to make further progress in *taijiquan*? Do I need to curb my desire?

The sensations you report indicate that you have already trained to the point where your *shen* and *qi* are substantial and you have internal power. Indeed, if you do not practice moderation in the realm you mentioned it will be difficult to continue to progress in the internal martial arts. Sex is one of humanity's strongest desires, so I'm afraid that it's not possible for the average person to utterly eliminate the *qi* of this habit. Might you be able to make a strong determination to eschew sexual activity and train assiduously for a period of three months, and thenceforth limit yourself to having sex once a month or once every two months? Of course, in addition to your own determination you need to also have your spouse's support. I never suggest forcing these things, as it would be unvirtuous of me to insist on anything that destroys the harmony of a family.

Master Ren, I have a question. If I am pushing hands with an opponent who also knows to gather and expel force from his or her waist, how should I "listen" to my opponent's insubstantiality and substantiality?

Once you have real skill, your opponent's insubstantiality and substantiality is not something you need to make an effort to sense. Your opponent's emptiness, substantiality, excess, and deficiency will all

---

[124] I directly translated the word this questioner uses, "勁路." I asked Ren what this means in person, and he succinctly replied: "The directions followed by strength in the body."

be as clear as day to you the moment you look at him or her. Only when an opponent's *shen* and *qi* are just as refined as yours are will you find it difficult to sense his or her flaws, while when faced with an opponent less refined than yourself there will be nothing that escapes your observation. Masters of internal martial arts thoroughly assess one another's skill the instant they make contact.

Master Ren, I would like to ask three questions. Firstly, do you ever practice a mirrored version of your *taijiquan* form in order to make your training more symmetrical? Secondly, do you think that paying attention to the breath and to opening and closing is a helpful way to reduce discursive thinking and enter stillness? Thirdly, please tell me whether or not the following statement is correct: when inhaling (closing), one should emphasize letting the chest drop while pulling the back straight; when exhaling (opening), one should emphasize straightening the waist and letting *qi* sink into the *dantian*. Please let me know what you think.

In answer to your first question, I have never sensed that there is anything lacking in the form that I practice, and I don't believe I am qualified to amend it. In answer to the second, all that is needed is to train until you have ample *qi* and *shen* in order for it to naturally become very easy to eliminate scattered thoughts. Having a stream of discursive thoughts means your *shen* and *qi* are akin to a thin object floating away. Finally, simply aim to relax and expand while you practice *taijiquan*—don't philosophize unnecessarily. Gathering and expelling are just gathering and expelling. They do not necessarily have anything to do with the breath.

Master Ren, please tell me whether or not I should intentionally guide the direction in which my *qi* travels through my meridians and channels when I am gathering or expelling power.

Please never under any circumstance try to guide *qi*.

Please explain how we should understand the notion of the body "containing five drawn bows." Also, if the body is like a drawn bow, how then can the waist be angled slightly forwards?

I have only ever trained in such a way that limitless bows are bent with a single draw.[125]

Master Ren, when I am performing some of the complex moves in the *taijiquan* form I train, I find it quite hard to keep my waist straight. Please give me some tips.

You need only maintain the sense that your waist is the force controlling and governing your body to be sure you are on the right path.

---

[125] The questioner is asking about an idea, common in the internal martial arts, which holds that a person's four limbs and spine should be like "drawn bows." I asked Ren about his enigmatic answer and he said he wholly rejects the "five bows" idea.

# 6

# Elucidations

*Some thoughts on traditional Chinese martial arts*

When the video of Xu Xiaodong and Lei Lei's arranged fight suddenly went viral in 2018, it inspired a large number of people to discuss and even attack the traditional martial arts, and some went so far as to mount an assault on traditional culture in general. Thankfully this furore eventually led to some fairly in-depth conversations about Chinese martial arts and the general state of traditional Chinese culture.

The various lineages of Chinese martial arts were all founded by people who experienced actual combat, developed tricks and methods for striking and grappling, and then trained intensely. Wildly distinct styles of martial arts came into being because their creators all had unique experiences, but whatever their differences may be, they are all devoted to learning how to strike an opponent with strength, effectiveness, hardness, and speed. While they may once have been formidable, in all honesty traditional systems and methods have been left far behind by modern mixed martial arts. Comparison under controlled conditions shows that in terms of strength, speed, and even technique, the effectiveness of mixed martial arts training is a world above what comes from traditional training with stone weights or heavy staffs. To cut straight to the point, traditional Chinese martial arts have not kept up with the times in terms of combat effectiveness because they long ago divorced training from real fighting.

Brazilian jiu jitsu is a traditional martial art, but the Gracie family established an academy that each year requires new methods to be extracted from members' fighting experiences at the same time as old techniques are constantly improved upon. As a result of the Gracies' research-oriented approach to real fighting, not only has traditional jiu jitsu avoided becoming an object of derision, it has in fact become a style that other martial artists humbly seek out in search of instruction. The spirit of these martial artists is something that we should all emulate.

I do know some genuine martial artists who are committed to studying and experiencing all manner of ancient, modern, foreign, and Chinese styles in their dogged pursuit of knowledge of real ways of fighting. They constantly improve upon themselves and cross the globe in order to try their hands against the best fighters they can find. As a result, some modern mixed martial artists have even arrived at my door to ask for instruction. All of this shows that there is a ray of hope that the traditional Chinese fighting arts will keep up with the times, but the people who really and truly understand the essence of the traditional arts are few and far between. Those who achieve themselves in the traditional way leave questions of speed and strength behind quite early on, as only in so doing can one find the place where the true tradition of Chinese martial arts continues to live. Those who worship speed and strength submit themselves to the limitations inherent in those two factors, and may even harm themselves in body and mind if they pursue them rabidly. After all, humans are subject to the laws of nature, and as such there are sometimes unbridgeable chasms between two people's capacities. If one's training, in effect, amounts to trying to develop the strength of a bull within the body of a goat, then the angel of death lurks close by. One need only look to the fact that many Thai kickboxers die young to see my point illustrated.

Now that traditional Chinese martial arts have lost the advantage in terms of training for speed, strength, and technique, can they still lay claim to any superior factors that modern mixed martial arts has yet to absorb? Indeed they can, but they lie in the realm of the so-called internal martial arts, which modern practitioners of traditional martial arts have more or less forgotten.

Let us examine *taijiquan*. Its name refers to using *taiji* philosophy as the basis informing one's approach to combat, to which the word "*quan*," or fist, refers. If this philosophy is used in pursuit of good health, then what one has is "*taiji* exercise," not *taijiquan*; if it is used in cultural pursuits, then the result should be called "*taiji* culture"—again, not *taijiquan*. However, nowadays there are a great many confused souls trying to use "*taiji* culture" as a guide for training in "*taiji* combat."

There are currently two major mistaken paths where *taijiquan* practitioners become lost. The first path is trodden by people who simply do not believe that it is possible to overcome an adversary without relying on physical strength; whenever these people lose to an opponent, they presume the reason lies in a lack of strength. For them, the word *taijiquan* is little more than a brand name plastered on the doors of their martial arts schools, and behind those doors they sweat away trying to build physical strength. Naturally, *taijiquan* practitioners are not especially good at strength training, and as a result they end up helpless in combat with those who are. Whenever this sort of *taijiquan* practitioner fights with a grappler he or she only has two choices: submit, or else completely disregard the teachings of *taijiquan* and start fighting just like a grappler. When they encounter boxers and strikers they are just as unprepared. Did Yang Luchan earn the name "Peerless Yang" by training this sort of *taijiquan*? Does the sort of art that only teaches you how to get into an awkward, tangled mess with your opponents have anything to do with the *taijiquan* upon which "a feather cannot come to rest and a fly cannot land?"

The second mistaken path is walked by those who cannot use strength but are at a loss as to what else they could use. They end up incapable of acquitting themselves even against the stragglers wandering on the path I just described above. Their end result is the sort of *taiji* exercise that is only useful as a healthy pastime for senior citizens.

## On "force"

Guided by the Confucian and Daoist teachings of "the universe and the individual merged as one" and "vast, rightening *qi*," the ancients realized that the ability of all things in existence to function as they do is primarily due to forces, and not the attributes inherent in any given physical material.[126] That a knife may cut the hand is of course because its blade is sharp, but the primary cause is found in the force that moves the knife.[127] Thus, provided there is sufficient force moving it, a chopstick can become a deadly weapon. In principle, then, even flower petals and leaves are capable of causing harm—it is this principle which underlies *taijiquan*'s thirteen forces.

Just like all other Yang style and Chen style *taijiquan* forms, the eighty-eight move form that I practice is no more than a methodology for training the thirteen forces. Force must be understood in order for one to have the ability to make real advancements in the study of Chinese culture and of traditional fighting methods. "Force" explains why, when young ruffians get into a brawl, it is not the biggest or strongest who prevail, but those with the most spirit. It explains why masters die at the hands of wild, untrained fighters. It explains why Mike Tyson could not be stopped, even though he was neither the strongest boxer, nor the most technically proficient.

---

[126] The first term is written as "天人合一" and the second is "浩然正氣."

[127] Force is from "勢," a character that can be found throughout the ancient Chinese canon, and which is also used as a component in a variety of modern Chinese words. I discussed this character extensively with Zhong Yingyang before he introduced me to Ren Gang. His understanding of its role in internal martial arts overlaps with the meaning of the word "force" as it is used in physics, but 勢 also implies power (in the sense of power in the human world) that is in use, as well as the forces (which may be unrelated to and far greater than humanity) that lead circumstances to unfold as they do. Perhaps key is that 勢 can imply that which has the potential to create change, as well as that which is already in action, creating change. Ren's mention of the role of force in the game of go in the next section is particularly illustrative.

There is an ancient phrase which states, "First gall, second strength, third *gongfu*."¹²⁸ Gall refers to force, strength to actual physical power, while *gongfu* is no more than tricks. Once a person knows how to use force, then strength and techniques cease to be of great importance. Knowing this means knowing that *zhanzhuang* is practiced to feel the power of steed and rider united as one. It means knowing that the forms exist only to help us practice maintaining the movement of force while the body is in motion. It means knowing that push hands and sparring are for learning how to remain cognizant and refrain from resorting to resisting with strength when under pressure. All of these points fall within the purview of a single goal: force. One who can use force halves the amount of effort while doubling the outcome.

A *taijiquan* practitioner who is still training strength and fighting techniques is better off just enrolling in boxing, wrestling, or mixed martial arts classes, as this practitioner has already embarked in a direction leading further and further away from what the wise masters of the past intended when they established this martial art. *Taijiquan* requires us to become adepts in the use of force, not to become strongmen. It requires us to be this way not just when we are doing martial training, but in each and every one of our pursuits in this world.

If you become a master of marshaling force, then strength and tactics will become insignificant to you. The jewel of traditional Chinese culture lies in this teaching.

## *The* guqin, *the game of go, calligraphy, and painting*

Among the praxes of traditional Chinese culture, the *guqin*, go, calligraphy, and painting hold especially important positions.¹²⁹ These

---

¹²⁸ In this phrase, which reads "一膽, 二力, 三功夫," the word "*gongfu*" refers to fighting tricks and techniques. But elsewhere *gongfu* simply means a high level of skill and achievement, including in "technique-less" training.

¹²⁹ The game of go originated in China approximately 2,500 years ago. It is called *"weiqi"* (from "圍棋") in Chinese but is typically known by the

four arts are some of the foremost tools for cultivating the mind. In calligraphy and painting, one's mental strength is trained via the mind's control over brush and ink. Once one's painting skills have reached maturity, one can wield a brush to subtly call forth whatever gorgeous scenery comes to mind. The more exquisite one's skill, the more one is able to take advantage of the shades of ink and shifting speeds of the hand's movements to portray the shapes and qualities of the ten thousand things.

The simplicity of the practice of calligraphy increases the demand for subtlety, as one's shortcomings are exposed the moment one begins writing. This is why most calligraphers practice for years before they dare hang their works on any walls. However, when calligraphers persist in practicing their art, as their mental power consolidates, they find that they develop self-mastery and the ability to remain unswayed by the distractions of the outside world.

Go requires players to remain in the state of constantly perceiving force. This awareness must not be lost, even when a match reaches the heights of tension. To sages and people of virtue, go was never merely a game to be won or lost; it was a tool for developing unshakeable mental focus. In the familiar image of Daoist immortals gathering to play this game, we can be certain they are not there to worry over winning and losing like mortal players.

The *guqin* is worthy of always being the first of these four arts to be named whenever they are listed. The practice of this instrument is a supremely marvelous way of bringing oneself into a state of deepened awareness. Even just quietly listening to the strains of *guqin* playing is enough to carry a person off to a very special place, but it is by "listening between the lines" that one may expand one's consciousness. This is why it is said that the *guqin* is not meant to be used for entertainment. It is meant to be used to pursue knowledge of self and to develop character. The ancients used the *guqin*, go, calligraphy, and painting to self-cultivate and nurture their original nature. These

---

transliteration of its Japanese name (written "囲碁," "围碁," or "いご"). The *guqin* (from "古琴") is a type of zither with seven strings.

pursuits give a person noble character as well as the ability to sense the ebb and flow of force as real life situations unfold.

It is no exaggeration to say that proper practice of *taijiquan* contains all of the benefits of the four aforementioned arts. In *zhanzhuang* and *taijiquan* forms, we use our minds to direct the forces of *qi* and the body as we perform each movement. This is an outstanding way to train mental strength, and it produces the same effects as learning calligraphy and classical painting. Pushing hands teaches us to keep force everywhere in our bodies instead of using our muscles or skeletons to resist an attacking opponent. This kind of mind training is very similar to playing go, but it makes one even more dynamic. When both people pushing hands possess similar levels of awareness, the one with more subtlety prevails by being able to simultaneously perceive both his or her own being, as well as the opponent's. The winner is the one who embodies the line in the *Treatise on Taijiquan* which reads, "Others cannot fathom me; I alone can fathom others." The practice of *taijiquan* pulls one ever deeper into the realms of subtlety.

*Taijiquan's* unparalleled value lies in the fact that it is an important tool for realizing the essence of Chinese culture. *Taijiquan* is truly a pursuit for the noble, and as such should not be mentioned in the same breath as those martial arts that were designed merely to hone mankind's instinctual fighting abilities.

## Taijiquan's *deepest teaching: Making use of emptiness*

Typically, martial arts ability develops through a process that goes from knowledge, to reaction, to feeling. Learning a martial art's "knowledge" means training so that the specific actions that the creators of the art developed become one's own bodily reflexes. After repeatedly training so that one has the ability to react in the prescribed way, one then moves on to "feeling," which means refining this reaction while actually sparring. The goal is to become even better at reacting in the desired way.

For those who have learned martial arts this way, one's opponents must attack in ways that fall within the scope of what one has trained to react to if one is to prevail in a fight. Furthermore, one's reactions have to be sufficiently accurate and swift in order for them to succeed. In reality, only a small number of relatively simple reactions can be trained up to the point of adroitness. If one is taught to train a hundred different reactive techniques, there will be no way to achieve mastery over any of them, and all one will end up with is a mishmash of "flowery punches and embroidered kicks." This is why it's said that you need only have truly mastered a single move in order to win most fights.

In terms of the course of progression from knowledge to reaction and into feeling, there is no question: the traditional martial arts possess no advantage over modern martial arts whatsoever. However, if we turn the discussion towards authentic *taijiquan* training, we see a different kind of progression, one in which the most important goal is the recovery of a certain state of awareness and the abilities that correspond specifically to this state. These abilities accrue from and are sublimated from awareness itself. They are not a form of habituated reflexivity based upon accumulated knowledge and training.

*Taijiquan* originated from the Daoist philosophical milieu and went on to spur an evolution in martial artistry. If the Daoist aspects of the training are eliminated from *taijiquan*, then it becomes training in musculoskeletal reactions in which *taiji* is nowhere to be found.

The most profound aspect of *taijiquan* is its clear distinction of *yin* and *yang*. To be able to distinguish *yin* and *yang*, the student must cultivate awareness and the abilities that flow from awareness, *not* knowledge and reactions. What must be trained forth is the capability to naturally perceive all objects and phenomena while in a state of motion, and to have the body be capable of spontaneously responding to what is sensed. The essence of this art is found in training to create these capabilities.

The above may sound excessively mysterious, but in practice it is quite the opposite. This sort of state is not limited to *taijiquan*—I recently discovered that it can be found in skiing, as well. If a skier uses knowledge to try and prepare the movements that his or her hands and feet make while flying downhill, this will only cause the skier to fall. To avoid falling, a skier has to enter into a state ungoverned by knowledge and analysis. From this state, a type of dynamism based on raw perception springs forth, and the skier's body constantly makes adjustments in accord with the terrain. This sort of perception has nothing to do with thought or decision making—it is pure awareness. The ability to instantaneously respond to changing circumstances on the basis of awareness is called *gongfu*.

Of course, what I just described can also be applied in martial arts practice. Yet it is here that we often bear witness to the misunderstandings so many people have with regards to how *taijiquan* should be trained. Specifically, their misunderstandings tend to center upon the word "*song*," which loosely refers to relaxation. Many people interpret *song* as simply meaning to slacken the body or slump downwards relaxedly. The flaccid way in which so many people train actually makes the body's ability to respond to changes increasingly clumsy, which is precisely the opposite of what the *Treatise on Taijiquan* describes with the words "a feather cannot be placed atop me, a fly finds nowhere to land." Relaxation or *song* in *taijiquan* is the state of dynamic, spontaneous responsiveness to change that is birthed by highly refined sensitivity. It's not what is typically meant when somebody heaves a satisfied sigh and says, "ahhh, I feel so relaxed right now."

Another misunderstanding lies in the way in which many *taijiquan* practitioners attempt to deal with adversaries' attacks by relying on analysis and calculation based on previous experience. This is not the optimal way to do things, as it never allows one to transcend the plane on which only those with the fastest and strongest physiques prevail in combat. The supreme approach will always lie in perceiving one's opponent using natural awareness and then responding on the basis of this awareness.

Skiing can be used to illustrate this point, too. While one skis, the ground beneath one's feet is constantly changing at a blinding pace, so if one attempts to predict and analyze, a crash is inevitable. In any complicated, fast moving situation, it's impossible to make calculations that take all factors into account, much less to keenly react on the basis of these calculations. Conversely, if one has reached a certain stage through proper training, then even in nerve-wracking circumstances it is possible to be aware of every fluctuating factor. If one's body is relaxed—*song*, not limp or flaccid—then it has the ability to remain poised in a state of responsiveness to all of the changes rushing through one's awareness. If one can ski like this, one need not worry about falling. In *taijiquan*, reaching this level of skill is described as the process of subtly transitioning from "the mind commands the body" to "the body follows the mind." In short, if one wishes for one's *taijiquan* to truly be useful as a martial art, this is where the path begins.

Today, *taijiquan*'s greatest enemy is students of *taijiquan* themselves, as they have destroyed Wang Zongyue and other predecessors' system for developing the power of awareness and the *gongfu* that corresponds to this power. What most people train instead are useless reactions. For instance, before pushing hands, practitioners think about the best ways to control opponents and to prevent being knocked over, whereas the essential teaching is clear: before pushing hands, one must let go of the ego and follow the opponent, as that is the only way to make use of this spectacular method for training awareness and the responsiveness that flows from it! This misapprehension of the core teachings is the reason that today most people use push hands to train a type of reactivity meant to prevent being knocked over. The fact is that this rigid way of training is utterly useless as a preparation for real fights, and that's why *taijiquan* generally seems to pale in comparison with other arts. The only way to win in combat with *taijiquan* is to appraise one's opponent's condition with lucid awareness, and then physically respond to his or her condition in accord with the principles of *taijiquan*'s thirteen forces.

Now, how does one cultivate awareness? The simple answer is that awareness can be cultivated at all times, not just during *taijiquan* practice or challenging activities like skiing. Zhanzhuang was designed in part for training awareness. However, one must realize that *zhanzhuang* does not mean trying to assume a low horse stance and hold it so steadily that somebody could balance two brimming bowls of water upon one's knees. This kind of training is ludicrous. The proper way of doing *zhanzhuang* is traditionally described as "having one's hands be like aquatic plants, one's feet as though standing upon empty space, and one's head as though suspended by a silken thread." This means that one's arms must feel like an empty, corked bottle floating atop water. The buoyancy thusly created then very subtly lifts one's waist, which itself in turn controls the rest of the body. Having one's feet be as though planted in emptiness means letting them seem to hang from one's legs. The instruction to feel as though one's head is suspended from a silk thread is also a reference to the feeling that one is standing in space.

The state of a person standing in *zhanzhuang* should be no different from that of a person soaring down a ski slope. One must be in control of oneself when practicing *zhanzhuang*, so one must gently lift the waist and remain sensitive to what the body is feeling. These conditions, when ripe, allow the thing we call awareness to emerge.

If one persists with practice, then the further one's *gongfu* develops, the more one will experience that things lying beyond the contours of the body can be made use of. After one is able to perceive the potency of the empty space surrounding oneself, there remain still higher realms to experience. For example, if one wishes to ski downhill on a black diamond course, merely making the body *song* will not be enough—the dynamic responsiveness that bodily relaxation yields is too narrow in scope and capacity to meet this challenge. However, if one can continue to *song* until the scope of one's perception comes to include the space around oneself, one will become capable of freely and naturally changing in harmony with the terrain. Keeping one's body balanced and staying in balance *with* the space one's body occupies are two entirely different skills.

Similarly, as one's ability to maintain states of acute awareness grows, the range of one's capacity for sensing and responding will also constantly expand. As this range expands, the energy one produces will increase. This is because any shift in space has the potential to act as a wellspring one can draw upon to create energy. This is why it is common to see true masters of *taijiquan* make only the slightest of movements and then send their opponents sailing away. To onlookers it may appear as though the master struck the opponent, albeit lightly, but what occurred was actually the result of the totality of the space occupied by the master and the opponent moving as one. The energy contained in a blow produced by the entirety of a space vastly exceeds the strength contained in a blow produced by an individual's musculoskeletal system.

Again, the more one's *gongfu* grows, the more it will be apparent one can use everything in the environment beyond one's body. The physical strength that comes from flesh and bones is very limited, but there is no limit to the energy in space. Thus, as one trains one will eventually return one's strength to emptiness, in return for which one will become a part of the totality of the energy in emptiness. This result is the true meaning of "refining *shen* to return to emptiness." In actuality, it means totally blending and merging with one's surroundings. This *gongfu* is also called "the individual and the universe joining as one."

# 7

# THE CAT'S MARVELOUS METHODS

*Original text and commentary*

I CAME ACROSS this story, "The Cat's Marvelous Methods,"¹³⁰ quite by accident, but when I finished reading it I was in awe. In terms of its author's level of realization, I would place it on approximately the same level as Wang Zongyue's *Treatise on Taijiquan*. This excellent story can be found in the Japanese novel *Sanshiro Sugata*.¹³¹ I hope that excessively nationalistic Chinese readers will not experience psychological discomfort upon hearing that this story comes to us from Japan, as the truths, artistry, and technique on display in this story transcend notions of national borders.

Regardless of where this story was first written, given how brilliant it is, we all stand to learn from it. This is how I understand "truth." Long ago I made a commitment that once I mastered *taijiquan* I would teach all people. So long as any person wishes to learn, I will teach him or her. The things I have learned in *taijiquan* cannot be learned by corrupt individuals, and yet if a corrupt individual were to somehow try to learn them, then in this process he or she would

---

¹³⁰ This story is entitled 〈貓之妙術〉 (*Mao Zhi Miao Shu*) in Chinese.

¹³¹ The name of the novel in Japanese is 《姿三四郎》. There is also a film by the same name directed by Akira Kurosawa. *Sanshiro Sugata* was written by Tomita Tsuneo (富田常雄) in 1942.

gradually become righteous. The martial arts, in other words, nourish people's essential natures. This is my sincere conviction.

There are significant differences between *taijiquan* and the other martial arts one might see displayed in public. Martial arts are not a shallow endeavor—they are a type of self-cultivation. *Taijiquan* is one of humanity's treasures, because anybody who practices it with diligence will receive great benefits at the levels of both body and mind. Only systems like *taijiquan*, which are guided by underlying philosophical principles, can embody the authentic spirit of martial arts. It is due to its philosophical background that in some regards *taijiquan* outshines the striking and grappling arts native to other lands.

One has to have real grounding in philosophy before one can access the internal aspects of *taiji*. Thus, the best thing a person who lacks such grounding could practice is not *taijiquan*, but rather the most pared-down form of fighting he or she could find. After all, the fiercest fighters will always be those who constantly apply themselves to simply learning how to kill. However, training like this brings one further and further away from the Dao, because it has the effect of increasing one's ruthlessness and one's animalistic nature, which ultimately worsens one's mental state. This is why we frequently see two major types of martial artists. One is basically without skill, and can only chatter about fighting or at best throw his students around; the other is overflowing with machismo and haughtiness, giving off the discomfiting air that he might even start attacking people at the dinner table. Neither type of practitioner displays the mettle of an authentic martial artist. My understanding of the way of the warrior is that those whose martial skill is impeccable exude a genteel air. Ironically, it is only accomplished scholars who ought to exude a touch of pugnacity.

The idea of scholars possessing something of a martial bearing is not one I present flippantly. For instance, it was the fact that he could not best Confucius in combat that initially caused Tzu Lu to respect his master. We might be prone to think that Tzu Lu, who was a military officer, would have been quite ferocious, whereas Confucius would merely have been a nebbishy man of letters. But it has also been passed down that Confucius was strong enough to lift an iron cauldron off of the ground. It is no surprise, then, that according to the Confucian ideal, a true scholar approaches the Dao via the pursuit of proficiency in ritual, music, equestrianism, and archery. The prowess that comes from such a regimen is not something that can be matched by those who merely train for raw strength or hand-to-hand combat techniques.

The above ideas are all touched upon in the following story. It may seem somewhat abstruse on first reading, in part because it was written in classical Chinese, and in part because it defies easy understanding by those whose insights into the martial arts have yet to reach a certain depth. Therefore, below each short chapter of the original text, I have added my reflections on its implications.

## Part 1

THERE WAS ONCE a lord by the name of Sheng Hsuan who possessed immaculate swordsmanship. One day, there came a great rat that wreaked havoc in his palace, night and day scurrying hither and tither, just as it pleased. Disgusted, the lord locked himself in his quarters and released his cat, ordering it to catch the scurrilous rat. The rat, however, showed not the slightest sign of fear, and just as soon as the cat pounced on the rat, it gave off a pathetic mewl and went running away in fright.

O, what to do in the face of such a scene? The lord went and borrowed all of the most valiant cats in the village and released them all at once in the palace. The rat was squatting in the corner of a room when it suddenly caught sight of this legion of hardscrabble felines. Without hesitating, it went on the offence and leapt towards them, and a ferocious scratching and biting ensued. The rat's onslaught was so violent that soon enough the cats were all cowering timidly, refusing to advance. The lord became so enraged that he took up his sabre and marched into the room to make a surprise attack, but not only did the rat dodge each fall of the blade, it began leaping here and there, causing the lord to demolish the palace's sliding doors and paper screens in his rage. Each time the rat jumped through midair it moved as fast as lightning and showed nary a hint of fear.

Of a sudden, the rat turned to face the lord directly, its face bearing the look of a bloodthirsty tiger getting ready to bite its victim. Sheng Hsuan broke into a mighty sweat and in desperation called out to his servant: "It is said that six or seven *li* away there is a brave tomcat of unequalled ferocity. Go and borrow that cat, and be back with it forthwith!"

Soon enough the servant returned with the cat under his arm, but when the lord laid eyes upon it he saw that it was a clumsy old thing with no sign of agility. But hopeless as he was, all Sheng Hsuan could do was try. He opened the door to the room with the rat just a crack and placed the cat inside. How could he have expected that the rat would suddenly freeze in terror, totally unable to move? As though it were the easiest thing in the world, the cat moseyed over to the rat, picked the rodent up in its claws, and gobbled it down whole.

---

The first part of the story sets the scene for a discussion of the highest levels of martial artistry, ensconced within the tale of a cat effortlessly catching a rat.

---

## Part 2

THAT NIGHT, ALL of the cats gathered in Sheng Hsuan's palace and asked the old cat to sit in the seat of honor while they knelt before it, respectfully asking: "We have all been studying the art of hunting for years, with total dedication to the way. Not only mice and rats, but even weasels and otters do we easily capture. Yet we never imagined there could have been a rat as mighty as the one we faced today. Honored one, we have no idea what sort of technique allowed you to so effortlessly catch it. Good sir, we hope that you might selflessly bestow your teaching upon us, and pass your marvelous skills to the rest of us cats."

The old cat laughed and replied: "You are all far too modest. Speaking sincerely, I can see that all of you already possess deep skill. It is only because you are not familiar with the principles of the Great Dao that you so unexpectedly lost in battle. Please, humor an old fogey and tell me about how you train and what kind of tricks you have behind your ears."

From the assembly of whiskered ones stepped forth a formidably muscled black cat who declared: "I was born into a family of rat catchers, and I diligently applied myself to learning this way. Since I was a kitten I trained in the skills of leaping lightly into the air, moving as fast as the wind, bounding over two meter walls, and even squeezing myself into mouse holes as small as bullet holes! I trained all of these skills to perfection, such that even when I am taking a cat nap nothing slips by me unnoticed, and I can wake up and pounce instantaneously. Even a mouse scurrying atop a rafter near the ceiling has no hope of escape when I am around. And yet! Today, defeat at the paws of this unimaginably fearsome rat has brought me the greatest humiliation of my life."

The old cat responded: "You train the way you do because you esteem movement, and therefore you are fettered by an overemphasis on grasping at your goals. In ancient times, those who taught movement required their pupils to first understand the principles. Even though their movements were simple, they were imbued with reason. Later on, people abandoned the principles and trained skills to the extreme, as they did not see the greatness of the ancient ways. When you have alacrity without a solid foundation and have a fetish for using little tricks, you will frequently exhaust your skill before you complete your tasks. The beginnings of self-delusion sprout from possessing a tiny mote of skill and relying on a shallow puddle of wisdom. You'll eventually hurt yourself with your little tricks and flimsy wisdom. You should all think about this three times each morning and night. Do your best!"

When the old cat tells all of the other cats that their skills are already quite established, he's reflecting the culture of wandering martial artists of old—when they won in battle, they still customarily complimented their vanquished opponents' skills. From this exchange we can see that the old cat was quite worldly-wise. But, in the end, it bested all of the other cats, so after it finished handing out customary compliments, the old cat told the assembled felines that none of them truly understand the martial arts.

The old cat's way of speaking was incredibly polite. I think that later on, if readers of this book find themselves wandering from place to place meeting other martial artists, they should make an effort to emulate such behavior. Having politeness is a must. In the martial world—especially when one is speaking about the older generations of masters—it is common for people to be merciless when they use their fists. But when using the mouth, there is always consideration for others' feelings. That said, I hope that readers will show a bit of mercy in both verbal and martial exchanges, as having restraint only in one realm and not the other is not particularly meaningful in modern society.

The situation nowadays is not what it once was. In the past there were too many people trying to make a living as fighters, and as such the martial world was fraught with danger. In those days, one couldn't operate under the assumption that everybody who knocked at one's door claiming to seek instruction was really what he or she claimed to be. Nor were challengers who visited martial arts schools always looking for a fair fight. In the old days, challengers might sneakily throw a handful of lime in a master's eyes and then start pummeling away, so extreme caution was necessary. In spite of or because of the dangers, civilized habits of discourse were a must in the era when competitions between martial arts masters were often a matter of life and death. In short, in martial society, elegant manners became so important because they were a way of demonstrating to others that one would not pull dirty tricks in the ring, or out of it.

All of the above constitutes the introduction to this story, while the real meat lies in what comes next.

The young cat who addresses the hero of the story describes what sounds like a terrifically rigorous and comprehensive training regimen, so why does it receive the "greatest humiliation of its life" from the wily rat? Think about it this way: if a martial artist were to tell you that he or she can jump five or six meters directly up into the air, take flying steps that cover a dozen meters, throw ten punches in a second, or even stand in once place with such a strong root that five or ten people couldn't push him or her over, would you think that this person has excellent *gongfu*? Well, this cat is akin to the type of person who spends all day in the training studio attempting to develop such marvelous-sounding abilities.

The old cat responds by saying that there are two levels of *gongfu*. The first, as above, involves the concentrated training of certain movements. For instance, in some martial arts people train to stomp so powerfully that they can smash a hole in the floor. Others train so that they can bash bricks or stones into pieces. Of course those are quite terrifying skills, but upon reflection one can't help but wonder whether or not they have much to do with actual fighting. In a fight, if one were to stomp the floor and create an ear-splitting cacophony one might scare one's opponent, but one would not likely land such a stomp on another person's body. Why, then, is this something that martial artists practice? What about if a person is able to stand immobile while a half dozen people try and push him or her over? Is that something that would ever happen in a real fight? It is hard to imagine an enemy approaching and saying, "Stand still while I see if I can knock you over!" Even if that did happen, all one's opponent would need to do is reach up and land a good smack on one's ear to get the upper hand. The training of these irrelevant skills has created an abundance of martial artists who end up with bloody noses when they try to show off their imaginary *gongfu*. Imaginary *gongfu* can be used in performances to show off strength, speed, and balance, but it is not practical if the goal is to become competent at fighting.

This kind of mistaken thinking can be seen illustrated by the fact that at least 90% of the martial artists in China believe that the point of *zhanzhuang* is to make one's legs and waist so strong that nobody will be able to push one over. Never do they ask a simple question: if this is so important, why don't boxers train *zhanzhuang*? Boxers never employ *zhanzhuang*, and yet there is little evidence that a Chinese martial artist stands any chance of overcoming a boxer! In fact, boxers train jump rope, which is quite the opposite of *zhanzhuang*, so why are they able to beat Chinese martial artists? Is the problem that *zhanzhuang* is a poor method, or is the problem that people do not know what *zhanzhuang* is really for? Was the experiential wisdom of ancient Chinese martial artists fraudulent, or have we modern people failed to understand it? To students of these arts, these should be pressing questions.

When the old cat said, "later on, people abandoned the principles," it was speaking about this sort of martial arts training. The old martial artists who lived centuries ago created and then passed on a large amount of theoretical knowledge, all of which was born of actual fighting of the most primitive sort. Each traditional martial arts move, each concept like "internal" or "external," and each mysterious-sounding training method was once something that the ancients developed on the basis of their study of real fighting. The problem is that if one does not really understand the knowledge that the ancient martial artists developed, and instead mimics the outer movements without knowing their underlying meaning, then the skill one will end up with is actually inferior to what one would achieve by simply training to fight in a very primitive manner. The prevalence of misguided approaches to training is a major reason that traditional Chinese martial arts are looked down upon by modern mixed martial artists.

Amid the readers of this book, there might be practitioners of boxing, tae kwon do, and karate who also find themselves being criticized by modern-day grapplers who think that such martial arts aren't practical. When this happens we should not blame the criticizers if the things we regularly train are indeed meaningless. If one daily devotes oneself to things like figuring out how to stand stock still while five people push and shove, then there is something very wrong with one's regimen.

Things go wrong because people do not follow the ancients' advice. Each time an ancient master created a specific movement there was always a reason for doing so. If there were not, he or she would not have created a new way to train. Only later did students of *gongfu* begin to gloss over the underlying reasons for practicing a method, and instead just blindly perform the movements. Please reflect upon whether or not that is how people now train. The predictable result of training like this is what the old cat described as "alacrity without a solid foundation and a fetish for using little tricks."

Take, for example, *zhanzhuang*—many students believe the horse stance is designed to create very strong legs so that one is impervious to losing one's balance, whereas in actuality this method existed to learn how to engage in armed combat while seated on horseback. The goal of training with this stance was to become capable of harnessing the force of one's mount's movements as a member of the cavalry fighting in war. A soldier who reaped the fruits of horse stance *zhanzhuang* training would have learned to merge his own body, the force of his horse's surging movements, and a large saber, thereby greatly increasing his deadliness on the battlefield.

Naturally, if one is practicing equestrianism, then one's body needs to remain relaxed, so that one will be able to flow along with the bouncing of the horse as it gallops. Were one to sit stiffly atop the horse, attempting to remain perfectly still, then after a journey of several kilometers one would be in agony from the jolting of the saddle. Thus, the very simple practice of horse stance *zhanzhuang* was created not to train leg and waist strength, but rather to begin teaching future cavaliers how to sense and follow along with the force contained in their horses' movements. The need to merge as one with the horse is why one must remain relaxed when practicing the horse stance, but even more importantly, this relaxation is also the first step towards learning to merge as one with all things.

I recall that in one of Wang Xiangzhai's books, he wrote that during *zhanzhuang* training he would frequently instruct his students to imagine that they stood facing a tiger or a panther, and to think about how they would grapple with such an animal. When Master Wang stood in *zhanzhuang*, to an observer it might seem as though he was merely standing still, but within his body was a sort of expansive force that never ceased its movement. By flowing with the wind, he allowed his body to manifest tremendous force. When he instructed others to do the same, his intent was to teach them to create force by moving along with the undulations of the wind outside of their bodies. The state of being able to flow along with the wind's movements is quite the opposite of the state in which one does not budge when a half dozen people are pushing with all their might.

The scolding that the old cat delivered bears repeating: "When you have alacrity without a solid foundation and have a fetish for using little tricks, you will frequently exhaust your skill before you complete your tasks. The beginnings of self-delusion sprout from having a tiny little mote of skill and relying on a shallow puddle of wisdom. You'll eventually hurt yourself with your little tricks and flimsy wisdom. You should all think about this three times each morning and night. Do your best!" I would say that this tongue lashing applies to at least nine out of ten martial artists today. Most people expend a huge amount of time and effort without ever realizing their aspirations. In fact, the situation is so grievous that it is not uncommon to hear about martial artists being beaten down by run of the mill hoodlums in the streets. I say this not to unfairly lambast martial society, but to squarely face the facts.

When the old cat says, "you should all think about this three times each morning and night," we should read this as an instruction to carefully consider whether or not the things we are training have practical applications. If they do not, then delusion has begun to infiltrate our regimens, and should we ever need to engage in real combat we will invite harm upon ourselves. So, should one determine that a method is useless, one should discontinue its training. If one is not sure whether or not a method would be useful in combat, then either one is training it incorrectly, or it is in fact useless.

To anybody who practices *taijiquan* but is still not sure what it really means to practice this art, I would say that he or she might be better off training the eight pieces of brocade *qigong* form. I say this because, if one does not understand *taijiquan*, then it will at best bring no more benefit than the eight pieces of brocade, and at worst might be inferior to following along with an aerobics program on television. Without understanding, the only difference is that a *taijiquan* form is longer, more complicated, and harder to remember than what is on TV. On the other hand, if one really knows what *taijiquan* is, then each movement and posture, each gathering and expulsion of energy, and each interplay between movement and stillness is an opportunity to directly experience the mysteries of *taiji*.

Martial arts training is only meaningful when one knows what one is doing and why. Without this awareness, any martial art is meaningless. One does not train *wing chun* to perform pretty movements—one should be learning things that can be employed in a real fight. If, after three years of *wing chun* practice, one still can't defend oneself against a thug on the street, then what was the point of all the sweat and sore muscles? Thus, starting from the most elementary horse stance training, one should aim to be very clear about why one is doing what one's teacher teaches. One should know what skill or strength each method is meant to develop.

Quite regrettably, most of us in the martial arts train blindly and confusedly; people who are clear about what they are doing are hard to find. I am sure that there are readers who have spent years of their lives practicing a number of different martial arts and yet do not know the purpose and application of all of the various movements and stances. I have a disciple who used to train with a very famous master, but he eventually discovered that he was only being taught to mimic movements. His teacher offered no instructions that work in combat unless an enemy conveniently walks into the movements of a memorized form. Ultimately the student concluded that this kind of training was pointless and he quit studying with his teacher. As far as I am concerned, his decision was a sign of intelligence. The scary thing is that there are people who train an art for a lifetime without ever asking themselves what they are doing.

Always keep in mind that the martial arts originated from people's need to defend themselves against adversaries—they didn't emerge from doctrine and theory. There are certainly different degrees of effectiveness and cunning when martial arts are compared, but the basic requirement is that they should be applicable in combat. If that requirement remains unfulfilled, then a martial art is not a martial art. This paradox plagues almost all of the *taijiquan* out there in the world today.

Thus far we have only discussed the first of the two levels of *gongfu* that the old cat alluded to. In a nutshell, the first level is where a great many practitioners of traditional martial arts find themselves. Practitioners at this level do not understand their methods' underlying reasoning, but they train their hearts out until they convince themselves that they are martial artists, even though what they are doing has no martial application.

The old cat broached the second level when he said, "even though the ancients' movements were simple, they were imbued with reason." In fact, the category he places ancient martial artists in is the same one occupied by modern competitive martial artists, including various types of grapplers, boxers, and mixed martial artists. Whether ancient or modern, all of these people train with very specific goals in mind. For example, nowadays some grapplers use heavy ropes or tires to train, but only to develop movements that they intend to use in the ring. Boxers may hit defenseless sand bags, but the real reason is to mimic the sensation of hitting another boxer in the flesh.

This is not to say that there are not numerous flawed modern training methods. As practitioners advance to higher stages, they inevitably discover that some of the methods they learned are ineffective or damaging to the body. So, they seek better methods.

If one is training a martial arts form that has students stomping on the floor each time they throw a punch, one would probably be better off just hitting a punching bag. One's opponent will land three blows in the time it takes to pointlessly stomp the floor in order to throw a punch. Stomping the floor is about as useful as trying to mimic Chinese martial arts movies where the heroes do double somersaults before throwing a kick. Anybody who has been in a real fight knows that fighting is extremely tiring. Most people are close to passing out after thirty seconds of serious fighting—even for somebody in great shape, there is no time for extraneous movements like stomping and cartwheels.

This is why I say that modern competitive martial arts are closer in spirit to what the ancient Chinese masters trained. The movements are always very simple—jabs, roundhouses, kicks, elbows—and all of them are readily producible in combat. The goal of a real martial artist is to be able to knock a person flat with one punch, not to memorize an eighty-eight move *taijiquan* form without having any notion what the moves are for.

However, here is the rub: neither of the two levels just discussed represent the pinnacle of traditional Chinese martial arts. Moving forward, the old cat gradually guides us further along in our ascent. His words are worthy of careful attention.

---

## Part 3

AFTER THE OLD cat finished addressing the black cat, a ponderous tabby padded forwards and announced: "I am of the opinion that in the training of techniques, it is *qi* that is the most important thing. Hence, I have specialized in *qi* for many years, and now my *qi* is so vast and far-reaching and brimming and strong that, why, it can fill all the space between the sky and the earth! When I face my prey, I first put the little varmint under pressure with my *qi*, and then I begin to attack. I listen to its breathing, pay attention to every sound it makes, and chase it left and right—however it moves, I never fail to adapt. Brilliance in using techniques and skills comes from having a placid mind. When the mind is placid, the techniques emerge on their own. And yet! This rat moved without leaving any traces, and I haven't any clue how or why."

The old cat presently responded: "What you train, verily, is ephemeral *qi*. That, in fact, is something that cats like me can conquer. It is definitely not the highest method. Here lies the reason: it is *you* who desires to trounce your prey, while your prey, too, wishes to trounce *you*. But, at the moment when winners and losers are decided, it is by no means always the case that the one who prevails is stronger than the one who submits. What you call 'vast,' 'far-reaching,' and 'strong' is *qi* that possesses form. Although it sounds like Mencius' 'vast, righteous *qi*,' in actuality it is something altogether different. Mencius' *qi*'s power came directly from *yin* and *yang*, while your *qi*'s having power is contingent upon an opportunity presenting itself. The two, therefore, are unrelated, and comparing them would be like comparing the eternal flow of a great river with a single night of flooding. So, when you encountered a wee rat whose force of *qi* did not bend to yours, it was still able to lunge and bite you, a hale feline, despite its being a weak little rodent. In that dire moment, with nowhere to slink or leap, of course you forgot everything and used your body to fight for your life. The rat's will was like a lightning bolt. How could your ephemeral little *qi* take control of such a potent force?"

---

This cat's *gongfu* is a bit like Mike Tyson's. In the film *Ip Man 3*, Mike Tyson squares off with the actor Donnie Yen, but it is clear that in reality Yen is definitely no match for Tyson—if the two of them were to have a real fight, there's a good chance that Yen would not be able to take even single punch from Tyson. Such a fight would be like a scrap between the black cat in the previous chapter and the tabby we just met. Mike Tyson is not a fighter who strongly emphasizes techniques, but because of the way he trained force, numerous other boxers fell to him less than a minute after touching gloves.

In terms of the force in his blows, Tyson surpasses 99 percent of the boxers out there. Numerous boxers begin each bout standing in something of a crouch and closely scrutinizing their opponents, cautiously keeping their adversaries at bay. Tyson fought differently. As soon as he touched gloves he moved in close, smothering his opponent as he rained punches. He covered his competition to the degree that they would feel incapable of throwing proper strikes, at which point they would succumb to fear and start punching wildly. There is an old phrase, "a single strongman can fight his way through ten trained fighters." If one has such *gongfu* that one's strikes are genuinely imbued with force, one renders ineffective all of the technical training and even the strength training one's opponent has sweated through for years.

The *xingyiquan* master Guo Yunshen was famous for defeating countless other fighters solely on the basis of his mastery of a single punching method from his martial art, called *beng*.[132] *Beng* is a supremely simple method—it involves no more than throwing a punch while taking a step forward. What explains Guo's prowess? Could it be that somehow his version of *beng* possessed some great, inexplicable secret? The answer is no—it was the *force* Guo could marshal that struck such awe into opponents that they couldn't even run away. When there is sufficient force in a blow, it doesn't matter whether one blocks it or takes it directly. In either case, one will be sent flying. There is no escaping force like this—when one's adversary possesses it, one's loss is more or less sealed before the fight even begins. Once a punch imbued with force is thrown, the chances it can be blocked are slim.

There are very few martial artists in China who use force. Instead there is a plethora of practitioners who devote themselves to trying to master this or that tricky move in the hopes of being able to best an opponent with it. One can train like this for a lifetime and have little potential for achieving any mastery, because there are no undefeatable tricks under the sun. Having a new trick up one's sleeve is somewhat analogous to growing a third arm and concealing it in

---

[132] Guo Yunshen's favored method is written "崩拳;" the martial art he practiced is written "形意拳."

one's shirt. If one somehow had a third arm, then one might be able to catch an opponent off guard the first time it shot out from under one's shirt to throw a punch. But there is no guarantee it would still bring much advantage the second time one tried to use it in that fight, and at any rate, once the secret was out, others would know to stay on guard for the extra fist. Special fighting moves suffer the same fate, so it is imperative not to waste mental energy trying to develop them. In both the internal and the external martial arts, true adepts' capabilities come from force, while the musculoskeletal system and specialized techniques play only a supporting role.

There are some internal martial artists who think that the goal of training is to create some sort of *qi* in the body, and then somehow get this *qi* to enter into an opponent's body to deliver a death touch. This idea comes from a total misunderstanding of ancient teachings. Adhering to it will only result in one being incapable of handling oneself in actual fights. However, if one rectifies this misunderstanding, then even the Shaolin arts can become internal. When one's understanding is accurate, there is nothing innately "internal" or "external" about any particular way of moving the body.

When the ancients spoke about *qi*, they were not speaking about what modern people usually envision when they hear the word. There are two ways of writing *qi* in Chinese, "氣" and "炁." The former, *qi*, includes the character "米," a grain of rice, in order to represent the nutritive essences that enter our blood after we digest foods. This sort of *qi* is what impels the internal organs to do the work of sustaining life; it is present in every living human's body and has no direct relationship with any form of cultivation. For instance, having ample stomach *qi* simply means that one will have a hearty appetite; having ample heart *qi* means one will have numerous worldly desires; having ample kidney *qi* will increase one's libido, and so forth. This *qi* activates the habitual behaviors that correspond with the various organs.

"炁," or *Qi*, derives from the transformation of *jing* into *Qi* in a state free of thought. This *Qi* also refers to the scope of one's perception. In *taiji* philosophy, *Qi* is synonymous with *wuji*. Represented graphically, it is "○," the circle from which *taiji* is born. In Daoist philosophy, both Qi and *wuji* are also synonymous with "the individual and all in creation merged as one." This means that if the heavens, the earth, and all between lie beyond the scope of one's direct awareness, then the sky is the sky, the ground is the ground, other things are what they are, and one is simply oneself. But, if the heavens, the earth, all other things and beings, and oneself are all encompassed by the reach of one's perception, then one is in the state Daoism calls "merged as one." The circle that represents *wuji* therefore also represents the scope of one's consciousness. Put in modern terms, this means that one's energetic field is just as broad as the extent of one's consciousness. The range of one's perception determines the breadth of one's prior heaven Qi.

When the old cat mentioned Mencius' concept of "vast, righteous qi" that fills all between earth and sky, that is nowhere not present, and that is enormous and supremely powerful, he was referring to Qi. This hearkens to a poetic Daoist saying, "To place your foot on primordial Qi is to roam through the great void."[133] The greater the strength of one's Qi, the more one will feel light, agile, and capable of doing things one never thought possible. This is why it is relevant to cultivation. In fact, if one constantly allows oneself to experience the full scope of consciousness—one's prior heaven energy field—then one will soon find oneself standing before the internal martial arts' gate of entry. From here, one will develop the ability to alter the movements of the energy in one's Qi field instead of directing musculoskeletal movements; this is what we refer to as moving force, which is the foundation upon which everything else in the internal martial arts is built. Consider the following: if one throws a punch, no matter how fast it is and how strong one may be, one is simply throwing a balled-up human hand. However, if one's fist is shot out as a result of the combined movements of force, the power of the punch will be vastly increased.

---

[133] From "踏元炁乎，游太虛."

If one tries to fight with a person whose force is much greater than one's own, one will be stricken with fear and be at a loss as to how to mount a defense. The feeling is much like that of finding a car suddenly bearing down upon oneself while crossing the road. It is not uncommon for people to lose their senses and freeze in place while the car is still quite far away. Sometimes people crossing train tracks become so terrified by the force of an oncoming locomotive that they stand motionless in terror upon hearing the horn and seeing the light of a distant oncoming train. The same happens to people who cannot find the wherewithal to run when standing eye-to-eye with a roaring tiger. In all of these cases, the victim is in terrible awe of the oncoming force, which comprises both prior heaven and later heaven factors.

The world is not lacking in people who are innately possessed of ample force, and they usually become powerful or influential figures. It is possible, however, for all people to cultivate more force than they were blessed with in the womb. That which needs to be cultivated is none other than the Qi of one's energy field. We have all heard certain people be described as possessing an extraordinary aura or bearing. What is described here? It is none other than a person's Qi field. This can be gradually cultivated by training so that one's physical body moves in response to the movements of one's Qi. These movements of Qi constitute one's bearing.

Instead of bringing it with them from the womb or cultivating it intentionally, many people also develop Qi in response to their environments and circumstances. There are countless rich people who believe themselves to be different from the rest of humanity and who fawn over themselves narcissistically day after day. Believing that they own the world and that their money is capable of solving any problem, they end up possessing gigantic force. Newly minted government officials might be terrified the first time they stand behind a podium to address a crowd, but after a few years of being fawned over and groveled at, they slowly come to believe that the people of the world belong to them. Their force, too, grows beyond what it once was, and they then stand before massive crowds with ease. However, despite their grandeur, both of these types of force are ultimately too flimsy to withstand any significant challenge. This is why plenty of politicians and rich people who find themselves facing corruption charges in court swiftly lose their gravitas and end up sniveling pathetically.

Returning to the theme of martial arts, I must reemphasize that training in techniques is inferior to training force; training external styles is inferior to training internal styles. Nevertheless, if one does not understand how to train internal martial arts, there is nothing wrong with training external martial arts. But the one thing that must be avoided is divorcing oneself from the realities of actual fighting while trying to think up one's own way of fighting.

Once one has mastered the use of force, all of the techniques, movements, and stances of the various martial arts will become dregs in one's eyes. Conversely, if one is still enamored with techniques, one's accomplishments are still only rudimentary. If one *can* use force, then one has truly got something—one has entered the door. Such a claim should not be made lightly, because mastering the use of force means being at a higher level than at least ninety percent of other martial artists. It does not, however, mean indomitability—at this stage, one may still lose. For example, although Tyson is capable of using force and few could stand up to him in his competitive days, so long as a fighter was able to survive an entire round in the ring with him, Tyson was likely to end up losing. This was because he could no longer muster his force in later rounds. Because he was technically inferior to most other fighters, he was destined to lose in a contest of technique and muscular strength. Feeling thusly cornered by Evander Holyfield, he became so panicked as to bite Holyfield's ear. One can never be sure that one's adversaries are ignorant in the ways of force. When faced with an opponent who has even a partial knowledge of force, there is no guarantee one's own strength will be able to restrain the opponent's.

The author of "The Cat's Marvelous Methods" was clearly a master who was richly experienced in actual hand-to-hand fighting. I say this because, were the author not a real fighter, he or she could not have so accurately identified the factors that determine winning and losing. Mere theoreticians can only paint in broad strokes—they lack the ability to point out the subtle yet crucial details.

The old cat's discussion of Mencius is both subtle and pertinent. It is impossible to be certain that one's own force will always be stronger than one's enemies'. I could potentially feel as though I possess such great force that I can encompass an adversary with it the moment we engage, but it could be possible that what I am feeling is something that has form. That which has form is not the same as the vast *qi* that Mencius alluded to. When Mencius spoke of vast *qi*, he was speaking of a strength, cultivated over a long period of time, that includes both *yin* (physical) and *yang* (spiritual and energetic) aspects. When one has this, one can at any time move the *Qi* that is one's realm of consciousness. Although he used the more common character for *qi* in his writing, Mencius was referring to *Qi*. This type of *Qi* is not impermanent; there is no time when it is not present. It does not come into being only when one decides to use force.

"Vast *qi*" describes the state in which *yin* and *yang* are harmoniously, naturally merged. Although it can be called into play at any time, that does not mean that when one is using it, it is then any greater or lesser than what it is at any other moment. The old cat compares this force or *Qi* to a river's eternal flow. In contrast, any force that is intentionally *created* is analogous to an isolated surge of floodwater. The expanded scope of awareness that one creates via cultivation and the corresponding force that one can then make use of are things that cannot be lost or diminished. Conversely, a contrived force dissipates into nothingness the moment an opponent parries it. Force created of *qi* comes one wave at a time. It is not the ever-present ocean that is *Qi*.

If one should cross paths with an adversary whose body is weaker than one's own but who is brimming with brazen assurance, even if one affects one's most threatening possible countenance one will fail to strike any fear into this person. Just like the diminutive rat in the story who is able to bite away at far stronger cats, such an adversary will be capable of going toe to toe with anybody. Particularly if such a person is pushed close to checkmate, he or she will find the means to rise to one's own level. In the ring with Tyson, other boxers always had the right to tap out. But if the rules of boxing were somehow changed so that each fight was a death match, one can be certain that plenty of fighters would have suddenly discovered they had the guts to fight well beyond their perceived limits.

There is an ancient story in which a general named Hsiang Yu punched holes in all of his army's boats and cookware to sink them to the bottom of the river he had just crossed before battle. By denying his men any hope of escape, he meant to demolish the timidity that can only take root in the heart of a person who thinks he has more options than just life or death. Life-and-death courage can be seen when a chicken rushes into battle against an eagle, or a cat fights tooth and claw against a dog much greater in size. This only happens when they have to protect their chicks' or kittens' lives.

The old cat's message to the tabby is that, when one is faced with an opponent whose life is on the line, any force and formidability that must be contrived into existence is of no use. One cannot strike fear into the heart of an enemy who is fighting to stay alive, and in fact it may end up being oneself who succumbs to terror when faced with his or her furious will to survive.

---

## Part 4

A GREY KITTY then lolled forwards with an easy gait and opined: "Elder one, what you say is very true. Even if one is overflowing with *qi*, if it has a form and leaves traces, then no matter how subtle one might be, this *qi* can still be sensed by one's enemy. I have long trained in the methods of the mind. I do not make sounds or strike fearsome postures, nor do I strive to be the strongest. I harmonize my body and my mind so that they become one. When my prey is stronger than I am, I marshal harmony in response, the same way a thick curtain stops a heavy stone hurtling through the air. I do not even need to push back when a strong gale blows upon me. And yet! Not only did the rat we faced today refuse to shrink before others' displays of power, it also paid no mind to my harmonizing. In the past my skills always worked divinely—I've never seen such a display as that rat showed today."

The old cat once again offered its thoughts: "What you call harmony is something you brewed up in your mind—it is not the harmony that just *is*. Even though you can dodge the sharp edges of your enemies' qi, you still have to create ripples of thought, stirrings which may be known to your enemies. When you focus your thoughts to force your mind into a state of harmony, there is impurity in your mental realm, and you lose vitality. If thoughts move in your mind, the feeling of spontaneity goes cold, and all marvelous effects disappear.

"But if there were no thinking and no doing, then even were you to move in response to what you sensed, your movements would be formless and unconditioned. What you would then have is the harmony that has no enemy under the sun—definitely not the useless knick-knack that you and those like you cultivate. When mind and technique are a single entity, each movement contains the ultimate principles. Qi flows through your entire body, and at the moment of opening, the paw moves precisely as the heart wishes, with no limits to its marvelous abilities. When harmonized, you do not use strength to fight back, even if you are being attacked with weapons of metal and stone. However, if your mind stirs even in the slightest, then you reveal your form in its entirety, and your *shen* loses its naturalness.

"That is why, even if an opponent's mind has not submitted, and he harbors the most antagonistic intents, no matter what stunning techniques he uses and no matter how hard it is to counter them effectively, I still respond naturally, with no mind at all."

---

The grey cat who appears here is no simpleton. I say this because it displays two major accomplishments. The first is its mind training. This cat has devoted itself to becoming capable of merging as one with its enemies. Secondly, it does not try to contrive force; rather, it senses its quarry's strength, and then regardless of how great that strength may be, it is able to transform it into nothingness instead of directly competing with it. Faced with this cat's prowess, most opponents find themselves powerless to respond. However, the rat in this story was not remotely phased by the grey cat, and the cat was unable to merge with it. In the end, this cat too lost.

The old cat's diagnosis of the grey's shortcomings contains a very important teaching. According to the venerable old kitty, the grey cat relies upon the actions of its mind to merge with its prey. The problem with allowing the concept of "merge" to form in its mind is that this actually causes the grey cat to lose its awareness and perception. The presence of thought makes it impossible for the cat to spontaneously come into harmony with its quarry in a state of full awareness, and therefore there is no way for its movements to flow in concord with its perceptions. This happens because, when there is thinking, awareness becomes stuck to thoughts and loses its keenness. When a fighter has thoughts, he or she takes a loss in terms of perception and the strength that flows from perception.

This chapter's discussion touches upon the highest realms of the martial arts. These are realms that can only be reached by a practitioner who has sloughed away thought and past experience and abides in the knowing awareness that exists by virtue of its own nature. Anything less than this keeps a martial artist trapped in the realm of reactivity. At the highest levels, a martial artist's state of mental-physical integration must be like that of a skier carving through the snow on a precarious slope or an acrobat performing on the high wire. Such lucid awareness can only appear when there is no role for thought to play. In the language of *taijiquan*, the name for this state is *song*. *Song* means relaxation, but it is *not* a state of flaccidity. It is also distinct from what is typically meant by relaxation, which means resting and relieving stress. The type of relaxation implied by *song* is what is done in order to elicit a heightened state of awareness. A practitioner's ability to be *song*, or lack thereof, is a key factor in determining whether or not he or she trains *taijiquan* correctly.

Requirements like these set the bar very high. In modern *taijiquan* circles there are masters who possess the agility of bullfighters and others who can fight like grapplers, but there are exceedingly few who know how to merge as one with their opponents. Thus there is little elegance to speak of when they actually fight. They might be able to dispatch with weaker opponents with a bit of finesse, but things get messy when they face stronger or faster opponents. This is because in their minds they still have the idea of merging with their adversaries, and their perception suffers as a result. *Taijiquan* teaches practitioners to "listen" to opponents' strength, but when opponents are stronger and faster, most *taijiquan* fighters' hearing becomes "muddy." This means that, because the opponent's body can move faster and exert more strength than the practitioner's own, the practitioner's mind, which is still governed by conceptual thinking, can no longer directly perceive the opponent's physical state, and instead can merely *guess* how the opponent will move. In the infinitesimal span of time in which a thought is born, the ability to flow along in spontaneous response to an opponent's movements is lost.

While the above may sound very cut and dry, I must emphasize that cultivating *song* is a gradual process. A *taijiquan* student must first come to experience the condition of being merged as one with an opponent. Then come the steps described in the *Treatise on Taijiquan* as "using the mind to move *Qi*" and "using *Qi* to move the body." At these stages, a student intentionally merges with his or her adversary, and then intentionally moves mind, *Qi*, and body.

After yet more training there then comes the stage called "the body can follow the mind." When one has reached this plateau, one naturally and spontaneously harmonizes with any person with whom one comes into contact, no matter what his or her inner state might be. Because of this, at the very moment of encounter, any would-be aggressor will sense that something is off, and will feel that something must be done to correct a certain sensation of weightlessness. He or she will feel like there is no way to throw a punch or level a kick, and will be left trying to find an opening. So long as one remains lucidly aware, then no matter how the opponent modifies his or her position, one's perception will be a step ahead, stripping the person of any way of getting a bearing. This is how an opponent is rendered incapable of making a move. A student of *taijiquan* methodologies must pass through this stage in order for him or her to transition from "doing" to "non-doing."

In this book I frequently remark that it is in the shallows of the martial world where one finds techniques. If one habitually wades in these shallows, then when one encounters an opponent who knows a technique that one does not, receiving a drubbing is inevitable. In the shallows, those who have more technical training defeat those who have less. In slightly deeper waters one finds *gongfu*, or skill. In these waters, one who is capable of mustering real power can trounce any number of opponents who are trained in techniques. Having *gongfu* fundamentally alters a person's body—a person who has it can cause grievous harm with a single punch and render others' best fighting tricks quite useless with very little effort. *Gongfu* trumps technical applications.

Further out from the shore, where the ocean begins to reveal its depth, lies rhythm. When an opponent can control one's rhythm, one's hopes of prevailing against him or her in combat just disappear. I saw a hilarious example of this in a video recently, where a hound was loosed upon a monkey who kept visiting a village to steal trinkets. When the dog went to bite the monkey, the monkey grabbed the dog by one of its ears and slapped it twice across the face, sending the canine running for cover. The next time the monkey was filmed ransacking the village, the dog refused to chase it. The dog knew it was no match for the monkey, even though it outweighed the monkey by several dozen pounds. In fact, even most humans who've never received any training would end up losing in a fight with a monkey. The moment an untrained fellow tried to attack it, it would snatch his glasses with one hand, yank his hair with the other, and put him in a terrible predicament. Even though he could easily kill it if he landed a solid kick, a monkey weighing only a couple of dozen pounds would run circles around such a man in a fight. Why? It possesses superior rhythm!

My teacher, Dong Bin, passed from this world when he was 87 years old. In his last years he was bedridden by cancer and became skeletally thin. Even so, speaking to me one day from his sick bed he said, "Ren Gang, if a troublemaker was to come in here, I would still send him running." That Master Dong could say this and be taken seriously was because his rhythm was incredibly fast. He said, "The moment the troublemaker moved, I would have already poked out one of his eyes and sent him running with a good smack across the face." Being able to run away would have been the would-be burglar's good luck. Because Dong Bin thoroughly understood the rhythms of movement, even in sickness he would have been able to perceive an opponent's rhythms and make it extremely difficult for the opponent to make a move. Even a deathly ill old person remains capable of using rhythm to overcome an enemy.

Past the waters of rhythm, once one is swimming freely in the unfathomable depths of the open ocean, one arrives at the apogee: merging duality into oneness. If one stood before a master with this level of ability, it would uncannily feel as though the master were moving one around. When the old cat chides, "if thoughts move in your mind, the feeling of spontaneity goes cold, and all marvelous effects disappear," it means that as soon as one starts thinking, one's perceptive powers necessarily dull. Thinking must cease in order for awareness to arise.

Pupils of mine frequently say to me, "It seems like whenever you use *taijiquan* it always works for you, so why doesn't it work for me?" The reason *taijiquan* still doesn't work for them is that they still react by doing—they still haven't learned to react with non-doing. There is no skipping the process of learning how to bridge the gap between these two ways of being. The old cat illuminates this point when he says, "If there is no thinking and no doing, then even though you move in response to what you sense, your movements are formless and unconditioned. What you then have is the harmony that has no enemy under the sun." Before one reaches this peak, one is learning *taijiquan*; once one summits the peak, one has mastered *taijiquan*.

When one's body does precisely as one's mind wishes, one is at last really doing *taijiquan*.

In response to these teachings, pupils sometimes express vexation and ask, "Do you mean there is no value in techniques whatsoever?" Naturally, techniques are not useless; the crux of the issue is that techniques that are not informed by the underlying principles discussed in this story are not especially useful. They are great for playing around with in practice situations, but they do not play a major role in actual fights.

For instance, I have a friend whose training in Wu style *taijiquan*'s thirteen push hands methods is very advanced. His most effective technique when pushing hands involves attacking from a side angle as soon as opponents stiffen in resistance, as a result of which his opponents invariably go flying in a whoosh. When I saw him doing this I had to admit that it was a really good technique, so I asked him to demonstrate the movements involved. A moment later we began pushing hands and I copied the technique he'd just shown me, thereby sending him hurtling down to the floor. Shocked, he asked, "How on earth can you see a move I've trained for years just once and be better than me at using it?" The key is simply that he trained the technique without imbuing it with the reasoning intrinsic to *taiji* philosophy, whereas I blend principle and technique as one. As one gradually absorbs *taijiquan*'s principles, one's techniques will work better and better, and one will be able to execute them with more and more finesse.

The thirteen forces of *taijiquan* that the ancients trained in all have practical applications. Conversely, while the Yang style form I train in contains eighty-eight different movements, one should *never* think that these eighty-eight moves can be practically used in a fight. *None* of them can be practically applied in combat. Rather, the eighty-eight different movements exist merely as tools with which to gain a sense for the contours of *taijiquan*'s thirteen forces, and then to practice working with them. Should one ever come to blows with an adversary, it is these thirteen forces that must be called to the fore.

Again, techniques certainly can be used, but it is incredibly easy for practitioners to become mired in the maze of techniques. Far too many students get lost on these winding roads and never find their way back to the root of *taijiquan*. Teachers obsessed with tricks and methods are countless. How many teachers have any direct experience with merging into oneness? How many students devote time and effort to seeking that goal?

In the story, the old cat acknowledges that the assembled throng of warrior felines are all armed to the claw with excellent techniques and methods, but emphasizes that they have yet to merge their techniques with deeper principles. Thus it declares, "When mind and technique are a single entity, each movement contains the ultimate principles, *qi* flows through your entire body, and at the moment of opening, the hand moves precisely as the heart wishes, with no limits to its marvelous abilities." However, I must make a point of saying that numberless *taijiquan* enthusiasts' training has been derailed by misinterpreting the idea of "*qi* flowing through the entire body." What this statement means is that once there is a degree of mastery, a *taijiquan* practitioner's body becomes a part of the prior heaven *Qi* that exists without obstruction absolutely everywhere. This statement does *not* mean that there is some special kind of *qi* flowing throughout the inside of the body.

The old cat nears the conclusion of this chapter by saying, "At the moment of opening, the hand moves precisely as the heart wishes, with no limits to its marvelous abilities. When harmonized, you do not use strength to fight back, even if you are being attacked with weapons of metal and stone. However, if your mind stirs even in the slightest, then you reveal your form in its entirety, and your *shen* loses its naturalness." In simpler terms, this means that once one becomes capable of harmonizing with others via non-doing, one will no longer struggle against any opponent. Even enemies who try to attack with blades or stones will be unable to inflict harm, and one will be able to subdue them. However, should one then begin to act deliberately, one will reveal something that is not formless to one's adversaries.

Lots of people, when faced with a strong-looking opponent, immediately start thinking, "I've got to keep this guy at bay somehow!" The moment this thought catches hold in the mind, one's body will begin reacting like that of a person who is trying to fend off another person. Therefore, one must always free oneself of thoughts whenever crossing hands with an opponent. Simply be aware of the other person, no more. This is the only way to cause an opponent's inner state to become readily apparent within the scope of one's perception. When one does this, a way of handling the aggressor will spontaneously and naturally appear. Learning *taijiquan* means learning how to fight like this.

The surest sign that one is sparring with a real master is suddenly feeling powerless to resist his or her attacks. When a *taijiquan* master gathers and then expels power, it feels as though one *forgets* to resist against him or her. This happens because, whenever a master enters into the state of moving in accord with his or her sensations, opponents can do nothing but slide into a bewildered state where thoughts of resistance find no footing. Were a master to begin a fight thinking about how to deal with his or her opponent, the physical state he or she manifested would reflect this mental activity and give the opponent something to struggle against.

How does a master manage to offer nothing to struggle against? It happens naturally. As soon as he or she expels force, an opponent will have already fallen into the scope of his or her awareness, and whatever body part the opponent was intending to use will seem to be floating in emptiness. This process is too subtle to be described with any eloquence; it can only be alluded to. My grand teacher used to use a simple simile as an illustration: "It is like a thief walking into an empty room." Imagine if one were a burglar, hunched over picking the lock on a thoroughly cased building, looking forward to making off with the gold, silver, and precious antiques one knew were waiting on the other side of the door. Then, as soon as one flung open the door, one suddenly found the room that was only yesterday stuffed with treasures now utterly empty, without even a single piece of furniture remaining! Undoubtedly, one would be so shocked and worried as to experience momentarily weightlessness. This is the condition that *taijiquan* masters create for their adversaries in combat. If one falls into it, one instantaneously loses all ability to wage conflict.

A *taijiquan* practitioner known for his skill in push hands once visited me for a bit of friendly exchange. When we pushed hands, as soon as we made physical contact I just spontaneously and naturally responded to him. Being a polite and straightforward fellow, he quickly expressed the unexpected anxiety he was feeling by saying, "This is bizarre—how is it that I feel like a novice who's never even done push hands before? I don't have a clue what I should be doing!" This renowned practitioner had never encountered an opponent who could remain empty. Typically, in the past, as soon as he applied any of his martial techniques, his opponents would reflexively react by resisting, thereby giving him a very easy target upon which to execute the rest of his technique. With me, however, wherever he tried to grab onto something solid he only ended up grasping at emptiness. As a result of my having merged into a single entity with him, he very quickly became unstable on his feet and started to feel that his body was in imminent danger. He could only keep expressing his puzzlement, "How come I feel like somebody who never learned how to push hands?" Students of *taijiquan* must eventually learn how to put others into this state.

Speaking sincerely, I do not at all feel that I have finished learning *taijiquan*. Each time I practice I am acutely reminded that the path before me stretches long, long into the distance. There is no false humility in these words. In the modern world, how many hours each day can most of us devote to *taijiquan* practice? Old masters like Yang Chengfu were not merely blessed by being born into families with intergenerational transmission of martial arts knowledge. They also trained with incredible devotion, sometimes unto the point of losing their jobs. To them, so long as they were able to train *taijiquan*, moneymaking was superfluous. Nowadays few people can choose to live like that, although some young readers of this book may still be able to live lives more like the earlier martial artists did. Those of you who do have such an opportunity, if you manage to truly understand the essence of the Chinese martial arts and then arduously apply yourselves, you will surely reap innumerable benefits.

One thing I frequently reflect upon is the fact that there is no shortage of people who study aspects of eastern culture such as Confucius, Laozi, and the Buddha's teachings. Yet, speaking objectively, how many of them can be said to have really received much help from all their study? Once, when I gave a lecture to a classroom full of successful entrepreneurs and executives at the Yangtze School of Business, I said to them, "All of you have certainly read Laozi and Confucius, and some of you are versed in Buddhism—you've read it all. But tell me, after finishing those books, how many of you really and truly changed? Are you just as greedy as you were before, or not? Do you lust after sex just as before, or not?" Nobody claimed to have undergone any real transformation. Is this because Chinese culture is useless, or because there was something wrong with the way they studied?

If, after reading through the classical Chinese canon, the only change in one's life is having something new to bloviate about while patting one's stomach after a long dinner, then one has studied in vain. This was where the dilettanteish executives and entrepreneurs found themselves after dabbling desultorily in the classics. Their problem was that they didn't study the right way—they tried to learn the essence of Chinese culture as though it were a form of knowledge that can be collected, whereas the reality is that Chinese culture is *gongfu*. In other words, the only way to cognize Chinese culture is through praxis. Once one has *gongfu*—real skill derived from actual cultivation—one is finally prepared to directly experience the things that Confucius, Laozi, and Shakyamuni spoke of. In contrast, not only is the intellectual understanding of classical writings that a reader without *gongfu* obtains fairly useless, it also increases the mind's propensity for deluded thinking. There is nothing to recommend in this kind of study.

One of the reasons *taijiquan* is such an outstanding art is that it allows practitioners to explore the praxis of classical Chinese culture. I hope that readers will find the way to directly engage with this cultural praxis via *taijiquan*, and that in time they will become conversant in the teachings of the ancients.

---

## Part 5

THE OLD CAT continued: "There is no ending to the Dao. You all must be sure not to think that my words touch upon the ultimate—be certain that there are cats shedding fur in realms far more rarefied than my own. Long ago, in the village next to my own, there was a cat that used to pass each and every day deeply asleep. Lacking even a pinch of vim, it slept as soundly as the earthen and wooden statues in our village temple, never once being seen pouncing upon a mouse. And yet! Wherever this cat slept, there was not one whiff of vermin to meow of. Invariably, each time it chose a new spot to nap, the rodents became just as scarce as they had been in the last location. One day I dared to ask the somnolent calico why this was, but it just blinked, yawned, and said it had no answer to my question. It wasn't that the kitty was unwilling to answer me, but as the saying goes, 'those who know don't say, and those who say don't know.' This cat had already forgotten itself, and forgotten everything else, too. Because of this, it had arrived at an incomparably marvelous state of being. The cat was no longer the type of rat catcher who relied on its strength and bravery. Compared with such a noble feline, I still have a long way to go!"

All along, the warrior Sheng Hsuan, as though in a trance or a dream, had been sitting off to the side, listening to the congress of cats. At last he found the temerity to open his mouth and address the old cat, saying: "I have long been a practitioner of swordplay, but never have I come close to the Way that you describe. This evening, by humbly listening to you cats' lofty discussion, I seem to have comprehended something of supreme importance for my path. Old cat, I hope that you will share more of your deep wisdom to further illuminate these mysteries."

The old cat replied: "How could I teach you anything? I am merely a mouse-eating beast who understands nothing of the human world. But, if you would allow me to guess, I would say the following: the key to swordplay lies not in defeating others. Rather, the true warrior is one who remains aware of the ways of life and death even in the most critical moments. You should steadily cultivate such a mindset before you train in the way of the sword. If you first become enlightened to the principles governing life and death, then your heart will be in no way skewed or imbalanced, it will contain neither doubt nor confusion, and it will lose its predilection for machinations and mentation. When your mind and your *qi* are harmonious, balanced, and empty of all things, then you will unperturbedly respond to whatever changes. That is what is called being 'present in the moment.'

"And yet! Should your thoughts stir in the slightest, then these principles will immediately escape you. You will become formed as well as conditioned, and then there will be both an 'I' and an 'enemy' to face off against one another in struggle. Should you fall into this state, then your marvelous ability to change will lose its freedom and its ease. If your mind thusly dies, and your alert brightness is gone, how will you calmly grasp hold of victory? Even were you to win, it would only be because luck was on your side, not because you understand the fundamental meaning of swordplay.

"When I say 'empty of all things,' I speak not of a dull, insensate mental state. Rather, it is this way: the very moment any being begins to gather power, its *qi* is already imbalanced. The moment its *qi* is marked by the slightest imbalance, it is impossible for that being to remain thoroughly blended with that which is vast and all-pervading. Once this has occurred, then if this being enters into opposition, it will go to excess; if it does not enter into opposition, it will suffer from deficiency. Going to excess means its *qi* spills away with no way of stopping. Suffering from deficiency means its *qi* is starved and useless. In either case, it is impossible for *qi* to expand

and transform. Thus, when I say 'empty of all things,' I mean that a being does not gather power, nor become imbalanced; it sees no enemy, and knows not its own self. At the critical juncture, it responds just so, without leaving any traces, and without taking any form. In the I Ching it is written: 'Thoughtless and non-doing, silent and motionless, one senses and thereupon knows all that occurs beneath heaven.'[134] I daresay that if a student of swordplay were to deeply understand these principles, then he or she would be quite close to the Dao."

Sheng Hsuan thought for a moment before quietly asking: "But what do you mean by not having any enemies and not having a self?"

The old cat purred softly in the flickering firelight and said: "If you have a self, then you have enemies. If you have no self, then you are without enemies. The Chinese word for 'enemy' once simply meant 'to stand face to face.' Whether you speak of *yin* and *yang*, or of water and fire, whenever things have form and appearance, then their opposites must too exist. My heart has neither form nor appearance, and therefore there is nothing that is its opposite. Only by forgetting the self and all other things can one truly be calm and untroubled. This is the only way to be in a harmonious state of oneness. Then, though an enemy may come into being, it is defeated before it even becomes known. Thus, without any thoughts, simply trust in your intuition and let it move you. In your heart be calm and boundless, and then the world will truly be yours. Do not become mired in your mind by the distinctions of good and evil, suffering and joy, or gain and loss. Though the expanse between heaven and earth is grand, there is not one thing outside of your own heart that is worth seeking. It is as the ancients said: 'If there is dust caked over your eyes, the whole universe appears narrow. When there is no dust left in your heart, your whole life becomes boundless.' It is most difficult to open your eyes when sand and dust are blowing into them. Metaphorically speaking, what happens to your eyes also

---

[134] From "易，无思也，无為也，寂然不動，感而遂通天下之故。"

happens to that which is fundamentally empty but luminous—the mind—when any 'foreign objects' enter into it."

The old cat allowed Sheng Hsuan to absorb these words before continuing: "Yea, though I tread on four paws through teeming hordes of a thousand enemies, even as my body is insignificant dust, my mind is still my own. Though my adversaries may be enormous, they can do nothing to me. It is as Confucius said: 'A general commanding three armies can be killed, but the wills of even the commonest of men can be unconquerable.'[135] And yet, were I to allow a moment of hesitation, then in that moment I would immediately become that which my enemies seek to slay."

As the assembly of cats and the entranced Sheng Hsuan listened quietly in the gentle glow of the fire, the old cat concluded: "This is all I have to say. You must all question and reflect upon yourselves. A teacher can do little more than pass on ideas and throw light upon theories. If it is your desire to seek the truth, then finding it is up to you. In Buddhism this is called 'mind to mind transmission' and 'a separate teaching beyond the scriptures.' 'Beyond' does not mean that this teaching contradicts the scriptures. Rather, it means that attainment always comes via transmission from one mind to another, outside of any written text. This is true regardless of whether a teaching pertains to the methods at the heart of Buddhism or to excellency in the arts. That which is alluded to in scriptures is that which is difficult for us to realize all by ourselves, and our teachers can only tell us to cognize these truths on our own. Thus, it is not easy to learn the truth from a teacher, either. Those things that are easy to teach and easy to learn rarely bring us into ourselves. In short, glimpsing your mind's nature—so-called enlightenment—means jumping clear of the realm of deluded thinking. This is synonymous with awakening."

At that, the old cat suddenly rose from its haunches, did an elegant stretch, and leapt onto the windowsill. Moving neither slowly nor quickly, it turned back to shine a Cheshire cat grin upon the

---

[135] Paraphrased from "三軍可奪帥，匹夫不可奪志" in *The Analects*.

whiskered assembly and its guest Sheng Hsuan, and then disappeared into the ink of the night.

---

The old cat's final instruction is for the listeners to take it upon themselves to reflect deeply upon the principles he presented. A teacher can clearly explain the principles, but in order for a student to truly comprehend the truths within, the student has to rely upon his or her own capacity for gnosis. That is called self-attainment. It is also called having an epiphany in the heart, or direct transmission from one mind to another. In any case, what is referred to is beyond words.

A teaching merely conveys the *questions* one is not capable of discovering on one's own. Teaching involves nothing more than a person who has already walked the path—a teacher—showing people how to comprehend things on their own. It is therefore impossible for a student to obtain anything by solely relying upon a teacher. It is not hard for a teacher to explain a principle, nor is it difficult for a student to understand what is being said. But it *is* difficult for a student to turn a teacher's state of being into his or her own state of being. If one's teacher has real achievement, doing so is called "recovering one's awake nature." It is also called "knowing the Way."

Restoring awake nature requires transcending all thinking and delusion.

It is also called "enlightenment."

# Real Taijiquan

## Afterword by Wang Xiaopeng

TAIJIQUAN'S IMPORTANCE FOR the future of humanity borders on the sacred. The mental realm that *taijiquan* leads to lies beyond both the impermanent physical human body formed by the four elements, as well as the illusory play of shadows that the conscious mind derives from the six forms of sensory input spoken about in Buddhism. *Taijiquan* slowly leads one into a place of freedom that brims with numinous consciousness—this is what the *Treatise on Taijiquan* refers to when Wang Zongyue writes, "I alone can fathom others, while others cannot fathom me. This is where peerless heroes begin." *Taijiquan* is a wordless dialogue between the limitless and the limited; it is a prophesy of future glory compassionately bestowed upon the miniscule by the vast; it is the power of the unparalleled mantra that liberates body and mind alike from the cycle of birth and death. Achievement in *taijiquan* yields more than simple valor and the ability to vanquish adversaries. Far more importantly, it brings equanimity, integrality, and harmony.

I came to know Ren Gang by way of introduction from one of my elders in the Ye lineage of *taijiquan*, Master He Jihong. One summer morning in 2012, I accompanied Master He to the Natural Path Academy in the Pudong district of Shanghai to listen to Master Ren deliver a talk on the *Treatise of Taijiquan*. I was shocked to find that the lecture was delivered with such eloquence and clarity that principles underlying *taijiquan* previously unknown to me were illuminated in a flash. I could see what *yin* and *yang* are, and how to embody them; I felt what it really means to let *qi* sink to the *dantian*;

and I could make out the nature of the relationship between *qi* and Qi! These three concepts alone were enough to upend the audience's preconceived notions about *taijiquan*. While I was shocked by the newness of all of this, I was also deeply moved by the sense that it was something long familiar to me. Perhaps this sense is related to what Buddhism calls predestined affinity.

I have now known Master Ren for over a year. Whenever I find a spare moment I try to pay him a visit to present him with whatever new questions about the inner meaning of *taiji* have arisen for me. Each time I visit, Master Ren kindly, sincerely, and patiently explains things to me in the most simple and direct terms. Never is his superb skill in *taijiquan* the only thing on display. Rather, he always leaves visitors with a strong impression of his humble and easygoing nature, his approachability, and his wise sense of humor. It goes without saying that I have received no small benefit from our friendship.

When Ren Gang demonstrates *taijiquan* he shows naturalness, strength, and softness in balance, which happens to be what is hinted at by the meanings of the Chinese characters in his name.[136] His *taiji* flows from his mind's nature, transforming so enigmatically that there is no way to clutch onto his truth. Anyone who personally experiences Master Ren expelling power will, in addition to being effortlessly propelled into the air, also feel marvelous openness and connectedness within his or her own body. This sort of magnificent power comes from the essence of one's being; it has nothing to do with what one might feel in the shoving matches typical of today's so-called *taijiquan*. Ren's power is reminiscent of a passage in the writings on *xingyiquan* that states: "When inspired power collides with your body, your world is turned upside down; this power meets enemies like the snapping of the string on a longbow."

Ren Gang is an inheritor of the Yang style *taijiquan* lineage that traces back to the almost mythically accomplished grandmaster Yue

---

[136] Ren Gang's surname, "任," has a number of meanings that are *yin* in nature, including "to let," "to allow," "to bear," "pregnant," and "silk thread." His given name, "剛," which means "hard," "strong," and "upright," is of a *yang* nature.

Huanzhi. Numerous notable contemporary *taiji* masters have publicly commended both his martial artistry and his character. Big-heartedly, Master Ren does not pick and choose students, and because of this he has given many people the opportunity to put down their poor habits and begin to study and practice the correct ways. In my opinion, this spirit is the embodiment of authentic *taijiquan*.

One thing Master Ren constantly reminds students is, "you must always be learning, but you also have to know *how* to learn!" In an age when traditional culture is slowly reawakening, at the same time as we carry forward the techniques of classical *taijiquan*, we must also constantly refine our characters using the teachings passed down by the sages and virtuous people of antiquity. Specifically, this means learning to embody the virtues of water so as to develop dignity and integrity. It also means mustering the fortitude represented by an image of water piercing through stone barriers one droplet at a time. Virtue allows us to be as attentive to detail as water finding and filling even the most hidden cracks. It allows us to be so at peace with ourselves that, like water, we take the shape of whatever vessel we may occupy without losing sight of our own natures. Virtue also allows us to compassionately render service to all needy people and worthy causes under heaven, just as equitably as the rain falls.

The publishing of *The Heart Treasure of Taijiquan* is a joyous event for the international martial arts community. This book will lead to widespread advancements in martial skill, inspire readers' hearts and minds, and contribute to the continuation of a traditional culture. This is not a text that a reader is likely to luck upon unless he or she is endowed with a certain amount of latent wisdom, good karma, and predestined affinity.

It must also be mentioned that Master Ren's ten years of research into the way of incense has made him one of today's foremost connoisseurs of agarwood. A thousand-year-old piece of agarwood continues to exude such soul-stirring redolence that a whiff of its aroma can silence the monkey-like mind and soothe chaotic passions. I hope and pray that, like agarwood, *taijiquan* will bring beauty and awe into the lives of all humans, and let us live as one.

In sum, may this book be a finger pointing at the moon. May it pierce beyond the merely apparent and reveal the ineffable truths hidden within. May it open students' minds and unravel all of their conundrums, so that each of us may move our feet and hands just as freely as we move our minds. All that remains to be done by those who resonate with this book is to carefully savor its words.

*Year of the celestial stem gui and the earthly branch si,*
*in Tongji*

---

Wang Xiaopeng is an associate professor and martial arts instructor at Tongji University. He is also an advisor to Longwen Confucius Society at Tongji University and honorary principal of Taichi and Mandarin Solutions in Canberra, Australia. He has won first place in international *taiji* sword competition and second place in international *xingyiquan* competition.

Master Wang, whose family roots trace back to Yongcheng in Henan province, was born in 1970. When he was five years old his parents moved to Mount Wandang (one of China's foremost centers of martial arts culture).[137] Starting in childhood he began training sword techniques with his maternal grandfather, who was also a renowned doctor of traditional medicine.

In 1977 Master Wang was selected to begin training with the martial arts team at a local athletic academy. He later began training the empty handed and weapon techniques of *chaquan* with Liu Xinfang, the son of grandmaster Liu Yuntian,[138] who was the first head coach for the Anhui provincial martial arts team in the early years after the communist takeover of China.

In 1989 Master Wang enrolled in the *wushu* department at the Shanghai University of Sport. There he studied Muslim martial arts including *chaquan* old fist, arhat's shovel, and *xinyi* two-sectional staff with Master Li Zunsi of the Hui ethnic group.[139] Later he trained long fist with the renowned *chaquan* master Ma Xiaofang. In 1993 he graduated and accepted a teaching position at Tongji University, while at the same time enjoying the good fortune of receiving instruction from the well-known Shanghainese Yang style *taijiquan* master Fu Zhongwen.

In 2001 Master Wang was introduced to the highly respected master of *xinyiquan* Bai Hengxiang, from whom he received precious further instruction. In 2008

---

[137] 皖砀山.

[138] The martial art *chaquan* is written "查拳."

[139] The martial art *xinyiquan* (often called "*xinyi*") is written "心意拳." The Hui ethnic group is written "回族."

Wang's connection to the Shanghai University of Sport created fortuitous circumstances that allowed him to meet and become a formal student of Master Jin Renlin, a highly accomplished inner-door disciple of Master Ye Dami. In the summer of 2012 the famous *taijiquan* elder He Jihong introduced Wang to Master Ren Gang, whereupon he experienced the nearly mystical wonders of *taijiquan*, which he realized flow from the very same source as the highest teachings contained in *xinyiquan*.

In 2013, entrepreneur Jack Ma and movie star Jet Li invited Master Wang to serve as an expert consultant during the creation of the "TaijiZen" curriculum, during which time he assisted in designing its movement forms. In 2014 he was invited to participate in the Conference on Collegiate Culture and Nan Huai-Chin's Pedagogical Theory.

From 1993 until now, Wang Xiaopeng has taught martial arts to undergraduates, graduate students, foreign exchange students, and members of the women's college at Tongji University. He strongly emphasizes that scholasticism and martial arts ability should be cultivated simultaneously, and that martial arts and meditation are one. He is the founder of a curriculum focused on the relationship between martial arts and meditation at Tongji University.

Master Wang Xiaopeng's writings include: *Movement and Stillness Combine, Yin and Yang Birth One Another—Martial Arts and Classical Botanical Gardens*; *The Benefits of Martial Arts Training in University Curricula*; *Applying Classical Thought in Modern Architecture and Landscaping*; *A Glimpse at Self Defense Study: Its Value and Inspiration*; and *The Relationship of Chinese Swordplay and Calligraphy*.

# The Shining Path

## *Afterword by Zhong Yingyang*

I BEGAN STUDYING the martial arts more than twenty years ago, as a little boy. Over the years I researched and trained in a wide variety of systems, including Shaolin, southern fist, *wing chun*, jeet kun do, eskrima, and the Chen and Yang styles of *taijiquan*. I always focused on learning the practical combat applications of these arts, and I had very little interest in the flowery and flashy displays of kicking and punching that are seen in performances. A fair number of ups and downs come to mind as I look back over the long years of my journey of study and practice. The only real constant on my winding path has been an undying urge to discover the true and real teachings underpinning the martial arts.

When I was very small in Hong Kong I was fond of training the spear and staff in my grandmother's garden, but when I was in my early teens our family set out for Germany. Although I suddenly found myself adjusting to life as a student in a totally foreign country, my youthful obsession with martial arts did not falter. While training in preparation for an all-Europe Shorin-ryu karate competition in which I later won second place, I also frequently sparred with practitioners of my own and other styles of martial arts in order to share knowledge, exchange ideas, and help us all improve our technical ability. Not long afterwards I was certified as an instructor of *wing chun* in Germany, and subsequently found myself frequently accompanying my more advanced martial arts brothers to train members of the police and armed forces. These experiences helped me to become adept at applying fighting techniques and built my confidence, but they failed to deliver real contentment. The feeling that I was far from glimpsing the highest peaks of the martial arts continued to nag at me.

In those years I frequently traveled between Germany and Hong Kong in search of various martial arts teachers, but I continued to feel as though I was wandering without a compass, and the bottleneck I had reached in my training resisted all efforts to break through. In an effort to cut through the Gordian knot in my mind I began reading voraciously, and slowly I caught glimmers of a simple truth that had long eluded me: the study of martial arts is not merely a question of moving the body. Deep study into the philosophical backgrounds of these arts is also required. By knowing the real meaning hidden within the physical movements, a martial artist has the opportunity to step directly into the eternal present. However, I also concluded that while books are useful, in order for an aspiring martial artist to break free of his or her chrysalis and emerge to float like a butterfly, a teacher who has already made it to the other side is needed to point the way. When I finally made these realizations, I laid down my books and told myself, *there is nothing left to do but wait patiently for the right opportunity to present itself!*

In 2003 I made up my mind to relocate to China, where I enrolled in Shanghai University of Traditional Chinese Medicine's five year undergraduate program. Outside of class I continued to scour the internet looking for a hint as to where I might find a teacher capable of transmitting the knowledge I dreamt of finding. I eventually travelled to far corners of China to study *taijiquan* with a number of famous teachers, and while they all had outstanding characters and martial abilities, I could not shake the feeling that they did not possess what I truly desired.

Finally, in the winter of 2006, my fortunes changed. That winter, thanks to a friend's unexpected introduction, I became acquainted with Ren Gang. My first impression of him was of a man possessed of both scholarly elegance as well as moral uprightness. He seemed to be a man with the reserved bearing common to masters of internal martial arts. However, I was still young and hot blooded, and on top of this I had a somewhat slanted view of *taijiquan*, so I remained very skeptical and approached him with something of a challenging attitude. In the midst of our first discussion, scarcely a sentence left his mouth without me interrupting to ignorantly make objections. Eventually, when he arrived at the topic of expelling strength, perhaps to give me a glimpse of his formidability, Master Ren demonstrated his point by applying a modicum of force to the center of my chest. Instantaneously, I felt his strength travel into my innards while a terribly unnerving sensation moved out to cover my entire body. Now *this* was something I had never felt before! As my shock dissipated, I quietly thought to myself, *might this be the teacher I have been searching for?*

Afterwards, with Master Ren's grace, I began to rigorously follow his teachings. The more I learned, the more I sensed the depths of his *taijiquan* skill. After a period of time I slowly came to see just why *taijiquan* is referred to as an internal martial art, how it makes use of *shen* and *qi*, and how practitioners merge as one with their opponents. *Taijiquan* as Master Ren has taught it to me has never simply been about the outward movements of the physical body, and instead has always revolved around learning to manifest the "*taiji* state." During my long search I had long ago read numerous instruction manuals and essays passed down by earlier masters of Yang style *taijiquan*; to my surprise I suddenly found myself capable of grasping their meaning. Not only did I understand their words, I was able to physically embody them in practice. These changes dramatically increased my faith in *taijiquan*. Later still, I started to understand the ways of nurturing "vast *qi*," of making use of force in order to train in transforming and expelling strength, and the ways of making the body equipollent, unobstructed, and connected. My body underwent a number of dramatic changes as my muscles and skeleton made adjustments in order to accommodate this new way of moving. It seemed almost as though a new body was replacing my old one, and all the while it became easier and easier to transform and expel strength.

Martial artistry aside, Master Ren has earned my deep admiration for his virtuous character. Over the course of the dozen years that I have studied *taijiquan* with him I have seldom seen him display any temper. His manner is always steady, optimistic, and encouraging; should his friends or students encounter difficulties, he always warmly steps forward to offer selfless assistance. This, I believe, is *gongfu*! Observing the way Master Ren blends *taijiquan* into all aspects of his life has led me to deeply appreciate that it is far more than a set of fighting techniques. *Taijiquan* is a philosophy that leads directly to understanding the meaning of life! Was that, in the end, not precisely what I had been seeking all those years? To have finally found it leaves me marveling in gratitude at my good fortune.

Zhong Yingyang is the chief martial arts instructor at the Natural Path Academy in Shanghai.[140] He began studying martial arts as a young child and has systematically trained in karate, Shaolin *gongfu*, Filipino eskrima, *wing chun*, and *taijiquan*. When he was 12 years old, he moved from Hong Kong to Europe, but he remained firmly committed to his passion. While in Germany he became the second-ranked champion in Shorin-ryu karate and was certified to teach *wing chun*. Destiny later provided a chance meeting with Master Nan Huai-Chin, who suggested that Zhong travel to China to study traditional medicine. Zhong later graduated from Shanghai University of Traditional Chinese Medicine and is now a licensed physician in China. After traveling around the country to study with numerous accomplished teachers, he formally entered the gate of Yang style *taijiquan* in Master Ren Gang's lineage.

---

[140] 自道靜舍.

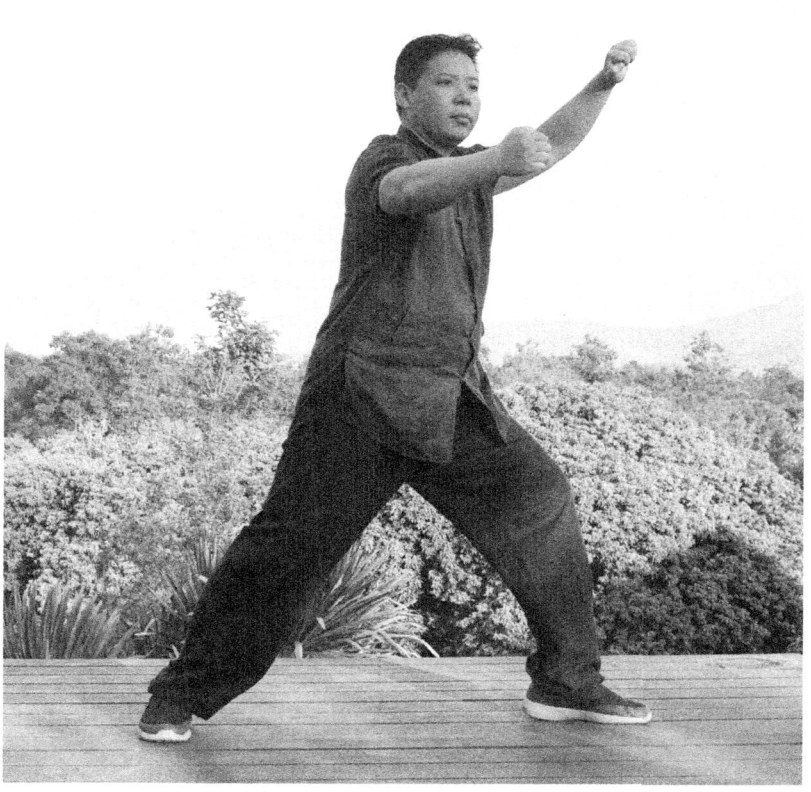

Zhong Yingyang

# APPENDIX

## Guide to Chinese Names Mentioned in the Text

Bai Hengxiang 白恆祥
Cai Guangfu 蔡光復
Cai Songfang 蔡松芳
Chang Zhilang 常志朗
Chen Changxing 陳長興
Chen Peng 陳鵬
Chen Qingping 陳清平
Chen Weiming 陳微明
Cheng Shubiao 程叔彪
Cui Zhongsan 崔仲三
Ding Ranqing 丁然清
Dong Bin 董斌
Dong Shizuo 董世祚
Dong Yingjie 董英傑
Feng Zhiqiang 馮志強
Fu Zongwen 傅鐘文
Gao Tieniao 高鐵鳥
Guo Dadong 郭大棟
Guo Yunshen 郭雲深
Han Qiao 韓樵
Han Sihuang 韓嗣煌
Han Xinghuan 韓星桓
Hao Shaoru 郝少如
Hao Weizhen 郝為真
He Jihong 何基洪
Hsiang [Xiang] Yu 項羽
Huo Zhenhuan 霍震寰
Jiang Fa 蔣發
Jin Renlin 金仁霖

Lei Lei 雷雷
Li Deyin 李德印
Li Yaxuan 李雅軒
Li Yishe 李亦畬
Li Zunsi 李尊思
Liu Xinfang 劉新芳
Liu Yuntian 劉允田
Lu Ban 魯班
Lu Wenrui 路文瑞
Ma Xianda 馬賢達
Ma Xiaofang 馬孝芳
Mao Zhai 茂齋
Nan Huai-Chin 南懷瑾
Pei Zuying 裴祖英
Ren Gang 任剛
Sheng Hsuan 勝軒
Song Shirong 宋世榮
Sun Lutang 孫祿堂
Tian Zhaolin 田兆麟
Tzu [Zi] Lu 子路
Tz'u Ming-Hsiu 慈明修
Wang Jurong 王菊蓉
Wang Xiangzhai 王薌齋
Wang Xiaopeng 王小鵬
Wang Xuanjie 王選傑
Wang Zhuanghong 王壯弘
Wang Ziping 王子平
Wang Zongyue 王宗岳
Wu Jianquan 吳鑑泉

Wu Quanyou 吳權佑
Wu Yuxiang 武禹襄
Xu Bingsheng 徐炳生
Xu Xiaodong 徐曉冬
Xu Yuqi 徐毓歧
Yang Banhou 楊班侯
Yang Chengfu 楊澄甫
Yang Luchang 楊露禪
Yang Shaogeng 楊紹庚
Yang Shouzhong 楊守中
Yao Zongxun 姚宗勳
Ye Dami 葉大密
Yu Hongkun 于鴻坤
Yue Huanzhi 樂奐之
Yue Tan 樂亶
Zhang Sanfeng 張三丰
Zhao Bao 趙保
Zhong Yingyang 鍾鷹揚

# Other Publications by Purple Cloud Press

2018

化性談
*Discourse on Transforming Inner Nature*
by Wang Feng Yi [王鳳儀]

Translated by Hausen and Akers

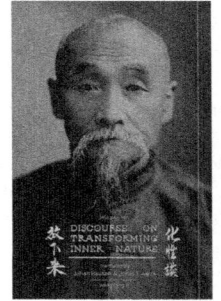

2019

經穴解
*Explanations of Channels and Points*
by Yue Han Zhen [岳含珍]

Translated by Michael Brown

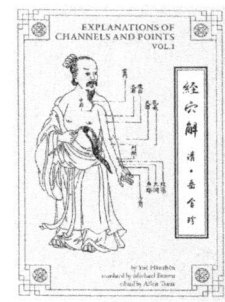

2020

太上感應篇
*Tai Shang's Treatise on Action and Response:*
A Commentary by Xing De [興德]

Translated by Hausen and Tsaur

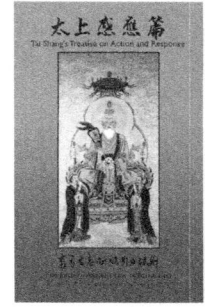

2020

*Path of the Spiritual Warrior*
Life and Teachings of
Muay Thai Fighter Pedro Solana

By Lindsey Wei

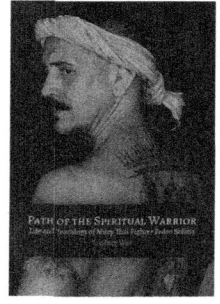

2020

景岳全書
*Complete Compendium of Zhang Jingyue Vol 1–3*
By Zhang Jingyue

Translated by Allen Tsaur

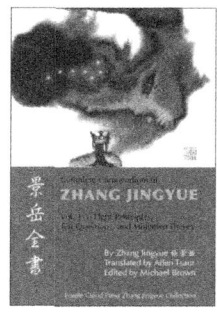

2020

修道四十九關
*The 49 Barriers of Cultivating the Dao*
by Xing De [興德]

Translated by Hausen and Tsaur

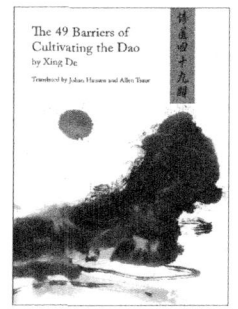

2021 (Forthcoming)

*The Valley Spirit*
A Female Story of
Daoist Cultivation

By Lindsey Wei

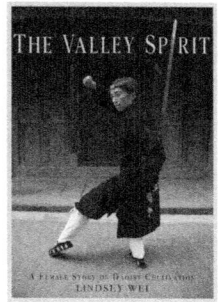

Printed in Great Britain
by Amazon